Available From the American Academy of Pediatrics

Achieving a Healthy Weight for Your Child: An Action Plan for Families

ADHD: What Every Parent Needs to Know

Autism Spectrum Disorder: What Every Parent Needs to Know

Baby and Toddler Basics: Expert Answers to Parents' Top 150 Questions

The Big Book of Symptoms: A–Z Guide to Your Child's Health

Building Resilience in Children and Teens: Giving Kids Roots and Wings

Caring for Your Baby and Young Child: Birth to Age 5*

Caring for Your School-Age Child: Ages 5-12

Heading Home With Your Newborn: From Birth to Reality

My Child Is Sick! Expert Advice for Managing Common Illnesses and Injuries

Nutrition: What Every Parent Needs to Know

Parenting Through Puberty: Mood Swings, Acne, and Growing Pains

The Picky Eater Project: 6 Weeks to Happier, Healthier Family Mealtimes

Raising an Organized Child: 5 Steps to Boost Independence, Ease Frustration, and Promote Confidence

Raising Kids to Thrive: Balancing Love With Expectations and Protection With Trust

Retro Baby: Cut Back on All the Gear and Boost Your Baby's Development With More Than 100 Time-tested Activities

Retro Toddler: More Than 100 Old-School Activities to Boost Development

Sleep: What Every Parent Needs to Know

Your Baby's First Year*

*This book is also available in Spanish.

For additional parenting resources, visit the HealthyChildren bookstore at https://shop.aap.org/for-parents.

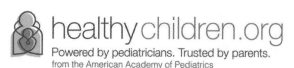

healthy children.org

Powered by pediatricians. Trusted by parents.

from the American Academy of Pediatrics

A 30-Day Wellness Transformation

Family
Fit Plan

Natalie Digate Muth, MD, MPH, RDN, FAAP

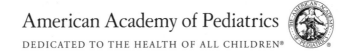

American Academy of Pediatrics
DEDICATED TO THE HEALTH OF ALL CHILDREN®

American Academy of Pediatrics Publishing Staff

Mary Lou White, *Chief Product and Services Officer/SVP, Membership, Marketing, and Publishing*
Mark Grimes, *Vice President, Publishing*
Kathryn Sparks, *Manager, Consumer Publishing*
Holly Kaminski, *Editor, Consumer Publishing*
Shannan Martin, *Production Manager, Consumer Publications*
Sara Hoerdeman, *Marketing Manager, Consumer Products*

Published by the American Academy of Pediatrics
345 Park Blvd
Itasca, IL 60143
Telephone: 630/626-6000
Facsimile: 847/434-8000
www.aap.org

The American Academy of Pediatrics is an organization of 67,000 primary care pediatricians, pediatric medical subspecialists, and pediatric surgical specialists dedicated to the health, safety, and well-being of infants, children, adolescents, and young adults.

The information contained in this publication should not be used as a substitute for the medical care and advice of your pediatrician. There may be variations in treatment that your pediatrician may recommend based on individual facts and circumstances.

Statements and opinions expressed are those of the author and not necessarily those of the American Academy of Pediatrics.

Any websites, brand names, products, or manufacturers are mentioned for informational and identification purposes only and do not imply an endorsement by the American Academy of Pediatrics (AAP). The AAP is not responsible for the content of external resources. Information was current at the time of publication.

The publishers have made every effort to trace the copyright holders for borrowed materials. If they have inadvertently overlooked any, they will be pleased to make the necessary arrangements at the first opportunity.

This publication has been developed by the American Academy of Pediatrics. The contributors are expert authorities in the field of pediatrics. No commercial involvement of any kind has been solicited or accepted in development of the content of this publication. Disclosures: Dr Muth reports a past financial relationship with the American Council on Exercise.

Every effort is made to keep *Family Fit Plan: A 30-Day Wellness Transformation* consistent with the most recent advice and information available from the American Academy of Pediatrics.

Special discounts are available for bulk purchases of this publication. Email Special Sales at aapsales@aap.org for more information.

Printed in the United States of America

9-405   1 2 3 4 5 6 7 8 9 10

CB0114
ISBN: 978-1-61002-338-2
eBook: 978-1-61002-339-9
EPUB: 978-1-61002-340-5
Kindle: 978-1-61002-341-2
PDF: 978-1-61002-342-9

Cover design by Daniel Rembert
Publication design by LSD DESIGN, LLC
Library of Congress Control Number: 2018964822

Contributors

Author

Natalie Digate Muth, MD, MPH, RDN, FAAP

Reviewers

Steve Abrams, MD, FAAP

Sarah Armstrong, MD, FAAP

Blaise A. Nemeth, MD, MS, FAAP

Staff Members

Debra Burrowes

Anjie Emanuel

Mala Thapar

To my husband, Bob

My children, Thomas and Mariella

Thank you for always being up for an adventure

Contents

Acknowledgments

Thank you to the families who shared with me their successes and challenges in meeting their health and wellness goals. A special thank-you to those who pilot tested the strategies, tips, and tricks that fill the pages of *Family Fit Plan*. This includes my own family—Bob, Thomas, and Mariella—who completed several 30-day family wellness transformations over the last few years.

I also want to thank my mom, who, more than 20 years ago, took me on an unlikely adventure to the Grand Canyon that strengthened our friendship and changed my life. That experience was the impetus for many choices I've made over the course of my young adulthood, training, and career. I'd also like to thank my dad, who showed me that when the time and circumstances are right, we can make changes that stick—even more so when we have the support and encouragement of our families.

I am grateful to the entire Publishing staff at the American Academy of Pediatrics (AAP), in particular Kathryn Sparks, who believed in this book and helped to usher it from an idea into what is in the pages that follow. Thank you to Holly Kaminski, who oversaw an editing process that greatly improved this book. Thank you to Drs Sarah Armstrong, Blaise Nemeth, and Steve Abrams, and AAP staff members Mala Thapar, Anjie Emanuel, and Debra Burrowes, who provided invaluable feedback and insights to make this plan most useful for families.

Finally, thank you to Dr Mary Tanaka for sharing her delicious, kid-tested, healthy, easy-to-make recipes that help bring *Family Fit Plan* to life.

Introduction

When I was 16, one of my favorite t-shirts sported the unlikely picture of a frog in a compromising situation. The stork, having just plucked the amphibious snack from a pond, found itself, instead of having a satisfying feast, being strangled by the frog. The advice below the image: "Don't ever give up." Who knew this shirt and its mantra would play such an important role in my life? This was the shirt I wore on the morning that my mom and I began a breathtaking and grueling 20-mile, 3-day hike down into the depths of the Grand Canyon, and back out.

But hiking wasn't always a part of my life. Through much of my childhood, I struggled to eat healthfully, sleep regularly, exercise daily, and cope with stressors in productive ways. My mom was in the same boat. Scared by the health risks associated with being overweight and inactive, when I was 16, my mom and I decided together to set ambitious goals to transform ourselves. We wanted to be healthier, more fit, and more confident. So naturally, we signed up to "conquer" the Grand Canyon—even though neither of us had ever even slept in a tent or trekked up a big hill.

My mom wisely enlisted the help of a personal trainer to help us get ready for our Grand Canyon experience. The trainer helped us develop a plan that would set us up for success. Week by week, we followed through on our plan, even though some days we didn't feel like it. Other days we wondered if we had made a mistake—why didn't we just decide to do something a little less difficult and a little less outside of our comfort zone?

But—*we didn't ever give up.* The pounding of rain on my face that late September afternoon, my whole body covered in dirt, 30-pound pack on my back, sweating all the way to the final step of the 4,000-foot ascent from the Colorado River to the South Rim, my mom right behind me, defined an experience that changed my life.

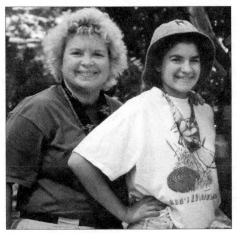

My mom and I accomplished something we could not have imagined doing even six months earlier. The trainer, who stood by us and guided and encouraged us as we set out to achieve our ambitious goal, launched me on my journey to inspire others. What started over 20 years ago as a lofty goal of hiking the Grand Canyon with my mom has led me to places and experiences far beyond my wildest childhood dreams—including a career as a pediatrician, nutritionist, and mom to two incredible and healthy kids. I am thrilled that the next step in my story is to share with you my Family Fit Plan.

The goal of the 30-day Family Fit Plan is to help you and your family kick-start your health and wellness goals and help you set the stage for long-term, lasting success in improving the health and well-being of your *entire* family.

The Family Fit Plan provides you with a road map, from getting your family on board to change to setting inspiring goals and taking the steps you need to ultimately reach them—all while improving the quality of your nutrition, fitness, and sleep and better managing stress and screen time use.

Special features interspersed throughout each chapter help bring your plan to life. These features include

 LET'S EXPERIMENT

These short activities test out the chapter's tips in a fun, "scientific" way, and allows a child to participate in an "experiment."

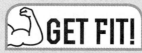 **GET FIT!**

Suggested exercises make it easy to incorporate activity into each week.

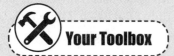 **Your Toolbox**

These practical applications help your family increase skills to translate a plan into action.

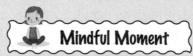 **Mindful Moment**

Suggested activities increase mindfulness and offer healthy ways to cope with stress.

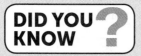 **DID YOU KNOW**

Surprising scientific facts help support recommendations made in the chapter.

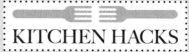 **KITCHEN HACKS**

These are quick tips for easy ways to eat better.

Recipes, activity plans and workouts, and online and in-print tools will help you take your Family Fit Plan to the next level. Most importantly, over the next month your family will have a lot of fun together on what I assure you will be an exciting adventure. There may be times that you will want to quit, but as I (and the frog on my shirt!) learned so many years ago, giving up is not the answer. Keep moving forward – even when it is tough. Not only will you successfully finish the Family Fit Plan but you may also have an experience that will impact you and your kids in a way that you never imagined.

Part 1
Getting Ready

Perhaps you want to achieve a fitness goal, such as finishing your first 5K or half marathon. Or your child has a newfound determination to improve his or her eating and exercise habits. Maybe a family member was recently diagnosed with diabetes or heart disease. Or you've come to realize that your family's habits around eating, exercising, sleeping, screen time, or coping skills need to be changed so you can raise an even healthier, happier, more fit family. Whatever the reasons that inspired you to pick up this book, the 30-day Family Fit Plan will help you and your family get from where you are now to where you dream you can be in the future, regardless of whether that is 30 days, 30 months, or 30 years down the road. Prepare for success by taking some time to get ready. Important preparations include:

1. Getting your family on board to join you in making changes
2. Understanding your family's starting point (baseline nutrition, activity, sleep, screen time, and stress behaviors)
3. Setting goals for your plan

Success Through Family Buy-in and Social Support

Deciding it is time to help your family boost health, fitness, and happiness is the first step in starting the plan. Creating a strategy to accomplish this is key. But first, consider

- Why do you want to start this plan?
- How much room do you have in your life right now for disrupting the old routines and creating new ones?
- Are you ready to go from wanting to change to making a change?
- Do you have family buy-in?

After you have given these questions some thought, check in with your family. I suggest you do this by scheduling a family meeting. If you commit to having regular family meetings, not only will you see better results from the Family Fit Plan, but you also get the added benefit of a stronger family bond, better communication, and improved self-esteem and problem-solving in your kids. Hopefully you are convinced that family meetings are worth a try. As you get ready to kick off your Family Fit Plan with your first family meeting, consider these tips for running an effective family meeting.

How to Run a Family Meeting

❶ **Consistency.** Schedule family meetings for the same time each week. Kids thrive on routines and consistency. If you have your family meeting on the same day and time each week, your kids will come to expect it and be more likely to participate. Choose a day and time and stick with it as much as you can (at least for the next several weeks). For many families, an after-dinner Sunday evening meeting works best to get ready for the coming week.

❷ **Keep it short.** Plan for your meetings to be brief—no more than about 20 minutes. Any longer than that and the kids (and maybe adults, too) will lose interest.

❸ **Follow an agenda.** Have a plan or purpose for each family meeting. Start the meeting by sharing the purpose of the meeting and what you plan to accomplish.

❹ **Set ground rules.** Ask your family members to help you set ground rules. Be sure to write them down. Sample rules include allowing only one person to talk at a time; considering everyone's opinion; and using "I" statements when expressing concerns (eg, "I am having a hard time understanding what you mean," rather than, "What you are saying doesn't make sense"). Rules like these help meetings to stay productive, upbeat, and positive rather than argumentative and frustrating.

❺ **Make attendance voluntary.** Encourage, but don't require, attendance at your family meeting. Try to make meetings fun so everyone will want to come, but don't force attendance. Some ideas to up the fun factor include playing music at the beginning and involving kids in helping to set and present the agenda.

❻ **Take notes.** Ask for a volunteer "scribe" to take notes for each meeting. These summaries will come in handy at future meetings.

❼ **Rotate the leader.** Take turns with who leads the meeting. This keeps it interesting and gives older kids and adolescents an opportunity to learn how to lead an effective meeting.

Your First Family Fit Plan Meeting: Getting Buy-in

Your first Family Fit Plan meeting gives you a chance to gauge how interested other family members are in starting a new health and fitness plan. Gather everyone together, and follow these steps to get a sense of who in your family is ready for your family wellness transformation and who may need encouragement.

✔ **Fun opener.** Start your meeting with a fun activity to help everyone get warmed up. For example, play some music to dance to, ask everyone to share what was the best part of their day or what they like the best about themselves, or start with a joke.

✔ **Purpose.** Share that the point of this meeting is to talk about starting a health and fitness plan. You want to see if your kids are interested in joining you to do it as a family.

✔ **How.** There are many ways that their involvement will benefit them. For example, kids who get at least 60 minutes of physical activity each day, sleep 9 to 11 hours each night, and engage in no more than 2 hours per day of recreational screen time score higher on tests of language skills, memory, planning ability, and speed at completing mental tasks compared with kids who don't. Only 5% of kids get enough activity and sleep and not too much screen time. Studies show that nearly 1 in 3 do none of the above. Maybe kids would be more open to trying to see if they could be in the 5%.

✔ **Why.** Kids and adults will be more fit and healthy. When parents are coached and guided in how to help their children succeed, the family succeeds as a whole. For example, studies show that when parents increase physical activity and decrease inactive (screen) time, reduce saturated fat intake, decrease exposure to unhealthful foods, change the home environment, and practice parenting skills, not only does the child benefit, but the parent improves health habits, loses weight, and decreases cardiovascular disease risk factors.

✔ **Complete a Family SWOT Analysis.** One way to see where your family currently stands before starting the Family Fit Plan is to complete a SWOT Analysis: a tool that businesses often use as they are pursuing new opportunities: a *s*trength, *w*eakness, *o*pportunities, and *t*hreat (SWOT) analysis (Figure 1.1).

✔ **Activity.** If your family is interested, choose one of the following activities to do together: What's Your "Why"?, "Best Possible Family," or "How Well Does Your Family Function" in this chapter. If your kids are not yet on board, close the family meeting by asking them to think about it because you would love for them to be a part of it. Also tell them that you as the parent are ready to make some changes, so they may notice some things at home that you control may be different—but in a good way.

✔ **Closing.** Close the family meeting by summarizing what you learned from the experience and list the next steps.

Complete a Family SWOT Analysis

As with everything discussed throughout the book, the best first step to making any change is to do a baseline assessment of where things stand today. One way to asses this is with a tool that businesses often use as they are pursuing new opportunities: *s*trengths, *w*eaknesses, *o*pportunities, and *t*hreats (SWOT) analysis.

Strengths include assets your family has that will help you be successful. These might include things such as adventurous eating habits, a routine of eating family meals, consistent schedules, strong supports, excellent sleep habits, or skill in cooking.

Weaknesses are challenge areas, or things that might make it more difficult for your family while you go through this project. These might be things such as very busy or chaotic schedules, dislike for exercise or healthful foods, food restrictions or very picky eating preferences, or inability or dislike of cooking.

Opportunities include things that might help you succeed with the plan, such as having a grocery store with healthful foods or a park or school nearby, access to cooking classes, or access to free or discounted membership to an athletic program or gym.

Threats are things that might get in the way of succeeding with your healthful changes. This could be a family member who is not on board with the changes or who may intentionally or unintentionally sabotage your efforts. It could be a disruption to the schedule, such as a job change, holidays, vacation, or change in season (eg, summer break).

Consider your family's strengths, weaknesses, opportunities, and threats while you plan for and implement your Family Fit Plan (see Figure 1.1, which is also available in the Appendix). This will help you make goals and action plans that optimize your strengths and opportunities, strengthen your weaknesses, and avoid or plan for the threats. You will refer back to your family SWOT analysis later (Chapter 3).

Figure 1.1. Family SWOT Analysis
List your family's strengths, weaknesses, opportunities, and threats that may help or hinder your progress over the next 30 days.

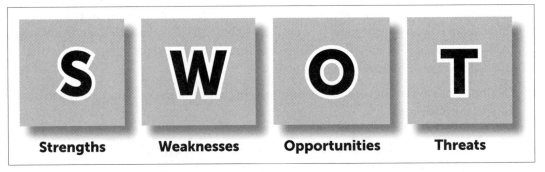

Activity: What's Your "Why"?

Why do you want to do the Family Fit Plan? The answer to this question may be different for each family member. By following the process outlined here, together you can come up with an overall guiding statement that will help you clearly define your family's "why." Knowing your individual "why" statements will help you tailor the plan over the coming weeks.

- **Make a list.** Ask everyone to come up with a list of what they'd like to get out of this plan. Ask each person to answer the question, "What do you hope to learn or do over the next 30 days?" Try not to censor or evaluate what anyone answers. For now, just add it to the list.
- **Identify themes.** Did specific goals or themes come up multiple times? For example, did a few family members mention wanting to eat better or find ways to be more active? Choose 2 or 3 themes that seem to be most important for your family.
- **Write down your "why."** Ask, "Why is this important to you?" Pull it all together and write down all "why" statements. For example, for some people it might be to avoid or treat a disease—"We need to eat healthier and be more active because we are at risk for diabetes, and we don't want that." For others it may be to strengthen family relationships and educate the family on what healthy looks like—"We want to raise our children to be

healthy, adventurous, and happy." Or perhaps it is to address a current crisis—"We all need to sleep better, eat without constant mealtime battles, and put some limits around screen time."

If your kids or other family members are reluctant, you can reframe the Family Fit Plan from a focus on nutrition, physical activity, sleep, screens, and stress to an adventure that will create opportunities for the family to try new things together: "It's kind of like an experiment. We can just test it out and see if any of the ideas work for us. If we don't like it, when it's done we don't have to keep doing it. Or maybe there will be parts that we like, and we can keep doing those things." Many kids will be receptive to this approach.

Activity: "Best Possible Family"

Envision your ideal, or "best possible family," by the end of the 30 days. This borrows from a concept in positive psychology known as your "best possible self" that helps to improve positive emotions, happiness, optimism, and coping skills.

Think about your family in the future. What is the best possible family you can imagine?

❶ Consider all parts of your family life—how you spend time together, schedules, behaviors, relationships, nutrition, activity, sleep, and stress management. What do each of these areas look like in your family's best possible future?

❷ Set a timer for 5 minutes. For the next 5 minutes, write about or draw a picture of your "best possible family." Focus on the future rather than the present or the past. The more specific you are, the more you will gain from the activity. Give extra thought to those areas in which you have the most control and where your actions can have the greatest effect.

❸ Discuss what each family member wrote or drew.

❹ Ask everyone to close their eyes for a minute and visualize your family as the described "best possible family." Envision a day in your future life when your family life resembles your ideal.

Activity: How Well Does Your Family Function?

High-functioning families tend to eat better, engage in physical activity more often, and spend less time sitting around. How well does your family function? Together, complete the General Functioning Subscale of the McMaster Family Assessment Device (Figure 1.2) to find out. Answer based on your family as a whole. Family members may feel differently than each other when answering the questions; however, you should do your best to come to a consensus for each question.

Figure 1.2. General Functioning Subscale of the McMaster Family Assessment Device

Mark the box that corresponds to how much you agree with each statement.

	Strongly Agree	Agree	Disagree	Strongly Disagree
1. Planning family activities is difficult because we misunderstand each other.	4	3	2	1
2. In time of crisis we can turn to each other for support.	1	2	3	4
3. We cannot talk to each other about sadness we feel.	4	3	2	1
4. Individuals are accepted for what they are.	1	2	3	4
5. We avoid discussing our fears and concerns.	4	3	2	1
6. We can express feelings to each other.	1	2	3	4
7. There are lots of bad feelings in the family.	4	3	2	1
8. We feel accepted for what we are.	1	2	3	4
9. Making decisions is a problem for our family.	4	3	2	1
10. We are able to make decisions about how to solve problems.	1	2	3	4
11. We don't get along well together.	4	3	2	1
12. We confide in each other.	1	2	3	4

Scoring

The questionnaire is scored by summing the numbers for each box you checked in questions 1 through 12. Then divide the sum by 12. Scores range from 1.0 (best functioning) to 4.0 (worst functioning).

If you find that there are areas for improvement, come up with a plan for how you might function better. If you find that there are many challenges, or it is difficult to come up with a plan to get along better, you might consider reaching out to a professional who specializes in helping families thrive.

Source: Used with permission by Epstein NB, Baldwin LM, Bishop DS. The McMaster Family Assessment Device. *J Marital Fam Ther.* 1983;9(2):171–180.

It Takes a Village...

Although your immediate family may play the leading role in helping to make and sustain changes, the larger social network that you turn to in helping you raise your family and care for your own mental and physical health is also important. That support can come to you either in person or online from many places—your kids' pediatrician; grandparents, friends, neighbors; religion, school, or work, for example. Nurturing and expanding these relationships, and trouble-shooting how to deal with challenges sometimes posed by a social network, can help your family make lasting change.

As the highly respected late pediatrician T. Berry Brazelton, MD, noted, "Families need families. Parents need to be parented. Grandparents, aunts, and uncles are back in fashion because they are necessary. Stresses on many families are out of proportion to anything two parents can handle."

Your Kids' Pediatrician

Pediatricians recognize the struggles and stresses that parents face and want to partner with their patients' parents to help a child grow up healthy and happy.

There are 5 family-level protective factors for a child's good health:

- *Parental resilience* (managing life and parenting stress and functioning well in times of adversity)
- *Social connections* (having healthy relationships with people, institutions, community, or spirituality)
- *Knowledge of parenting and child development* (implementing developmentally appropriate best parenting practices)
- *Concrete support in times of need* (identifying, accessing, advocating for, and receiving needed services to promote healthy development)
- *Social and emotional competence of children* (providing an environment and experiences that help children develop close and secure relationships and learn to regulate and express emotions in a productive way)

Pediatricians are increasingly well versed in these factors and can help you identify your strengths and provide you with tools and resources to help you improve.

One way to tap into the pediatrician's experience as a part of your village is to come to well-child visits (also known as health supervision visits) with a plan to get the most out of your time together. Your child's growth, development, nutrition, activity, screen time, sleep, and behavior are monitored at every well-child visit, which should occur annually for children 3 years and older and more frequently for children younger than 3 years (generally at birth, age 2 to 4 weeks, and at 2, 4, 6, 9, 12, 15, 18, 24, and 30 months). Consider answering the questions in the previsit checklist in Figure 1.3 (and in the Appendix) before your next visit. Even if you don't bring this list with you to the visit, it helps you to get a sense of what is going well and where you might have questions that the pediatrician can help answer.

Figure 1.3. Previsit Checklist

Adapted from the American Academy of Pediatrics Bright Futures clinician and family resources, this previsit checklist can help you focus on those topics you find to be most important and also note those areas where you feel you do well as a parent. Consider filling out this checklist before your child's next well-child visit to help make sure you leave the visit with the tools and resources you need to help your child and family thrive. Note that the checklist is adapted to focus only on those items relevant to your Family Fit Plan.

	Things I Do Well as a Parent	Things I Would Like to Discuss Today
Feeding my child		
Understanding what to expect next from my child		
Managing my child's behavior		
Helping my child sleep		
Using resources in my community to help my child		
Helping my child fit into our family; get along with others		
Helping my family handle stress		
Helping my child learn through play and be physically active		
Managing my child's moods		
Managing my child's screen time		
Setting routines		

Source: Adapted from American Academy of Pediatrics. *Bright Futures: Nutrition.* Elk Grove Village, IL: American Academy of Pediatrics; 2011.

When you are at the visit, ask to see your child's growth chart, and ask for your pediatrician's interpretation of the height, weight, and body mass index (BMI) percentile curves (or weight-for-length percentile for kids younger than 2 years). Each of these curves provides significant information about your child's health.

Height curve: After about age 3 years, a child's height tends to track along a fairly consistent height percentile. As a rule of thumb, you can expect your boy's height as an adult to be (mom's height [inches] + 5 inches + dad's height [inches]/2 and your girl's height as an adult to be (mom's height [inches] + dad's height [inches] – 5 inches)/2 plus or minus a couple of inches.

Weight curve: A child's weight is affected by many factors, but most often weight concerns are due to too little or too much caloric intake. A pediatrician will track your child's weight gain to try to identify early on if there are concerns in too little or too much gain from year to year.

Figure 1.4 shows growth and weight changes you can expect based on your child's age and stage of development.

Figure 1.4. Expected Growth by Age and Stage

	Growth	Weight	Key Considerations
Infant (0 months to 12 months)	50% increase from birth length by age 1 year	Initial weight loss, then back to birth weight by age 2 weeks Then gain about 1 lb every 2 weeks Double birth weight by age 4 to 6 months. Triple by age 1.	
Toddler and Preschooler (1 year to 4 years)	2½ to 3½ inches per year	4½ to 6½ lb gain per year	
School Aged (5 years to 10 Years)	2½ inches per year	7 lb gain per year	
Adolescent (11 years to 18 Years)	4½ inches per year at onset of puberty. Overall, gain last 15% to 20% of adult height. Females stop growing within 2 years after first menstrual period.	Gain 50% of final adult weight during these years.	Females gain fat in hips, thighs, and buttocks. Normal to go from 15% to 18% body fat prior to puberty to 20% to 25% after puberty. Males gain weight before the growth spurt at ages 9 to 13 years when body fat percentage decreases. Body fat increases after puberty to an adult norm of 15% to 18% body fat.

Source: American Academy of Pediatrics. *Bright Futures: Nutrition*. Elk Grove Village, IL: American Academy of Pediatrics; 2011.

Body mass index percentile: Body mass index is a measure of height and weight. The formula for BMI is weight (in kilograms) divided by height (in meters) squared. The formula is used as a way of estimating a person's body fat. For adults, the BMI number helps to indicate health risk. An adult with a BMI greater than 25 is considered to be overweight, while those with a BMI greater than 30 are considered to have obesity. Because children are continually growing and experience spurts at certain ages (eg, a typical child will have a decrease in BMI around 4 years and then progressively increase throughout childhood), BMI percentile is plotted on an age- and gender-appropriate growth chart to assess if the child is at a healthy weight (Figure 1.5).

Figure 1.5. Body Mass Index Percentile: What It Means

The following is an example of how sample body mass index (BMI) numbers would be interpreted for a 10-year-old boy:

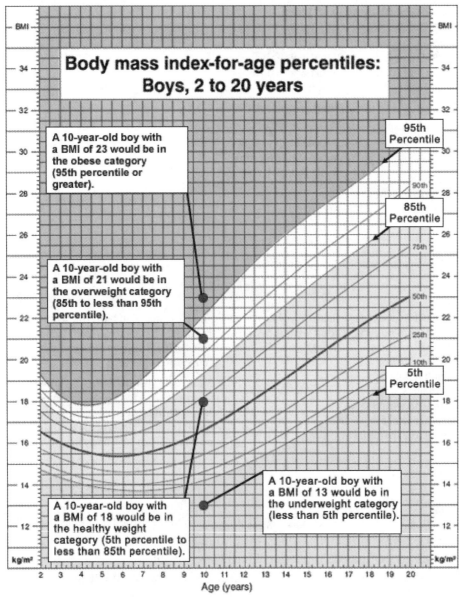

Source: Centers for Disease Control and Prevention. https://www.cdc.gov/healthyweight/assessing/bmi/childrens_bmi/about_childrens_bmi.html. Accessed March 19, 2019.

Once you know a child's height and weight, you can figure out the BMI percentile using a calculator such as the one available through the Centers for Disease Control and Prevention at https://www.cdc.gov/healthyweight/bmi/calculator.html. Body mass index is a good estimate of body fat, but it is not a perfect measure. It may overestimate fat in muscular individuals and underestimate fat in individuals with normal weight but a high percentage of body fat compared with muscle. Still, it offers a pretty good idea of whether to be concerned about your child's weight.

Be prepared for your child's pediatrician to discuss height, weight, and BMI. Before the visit, have a conversation with your child about what will occur at the appointment, including measuring height and weight.

If you worry that your child may not be at a healthy weight, discuss this sensitively with your child. Avoid words like "fat," "diet," and "obese." Instead, focus on being healthy. Weight is only one piece of a much bigger picture. Behaviors like eating healthy, being active, getting enough sleep at night, managing stress in a positive way, and avoiding too much screen time play a more important role.

Plan in advance of the appointment how you would like to talk about weight with your child's pediatrician and how you would like your pediatrician to best support you and your child. Based on your child's growth chart, the pediatrician may recommend further tests if there are concerns about your child's height, weight, or BMI percentile, or if there is risk or signs of other health issues.

Often, pediatricians are well connected to community resources, and if you share that you are working on improving your family's overall fitness, especially in the areas of nutrition, physical activity, sleep, stress management, and screen time, your child's pediatrician may be able to direct you to community resources and tools that can help you keep up your plan.

The American Academy of Pediatrics book *Achieving a Healthy Weight for Your Child: An Action Plan for Families,* by Sandra G. Hassink, MD, MS, FAAP, is an excellent resource to learn more about how to talk to your child and your child's pediatrician about weight. In addition, many tools are available to help you further prepare for your visit to the pediatrician, such as the Well-Visit Planner (https://www.wellvisitplanner.org/education and https://www.wellvisitplanner.org/questionnaire) and the Agency for Healthcare Research and Quality patient question builder (https://www.ahrq.gov/patients-consumers/question-builder.html).

Grandparents

One of the most important relationships to navigate as you plan to turn your Family Fit Plan into a way of life is the relationship with your parents and in-laws, because they may be able to support you. After all, both parents and grandparents want the kids to be happy and healthy. However, grandparents often consider one of their main roles to be to spoil their grandchildren, and much of the time this comes in the form of food—and lots of it. Some grandparents may have a bit of a defiant toddler streak in them—the more you tell them they cannot do what they see as one of their key functions, the more likely they are to do it. As comedian Sam Levenson said in jest, "The reason grandparents and grandchildren get along so well is that they have a common enemy." If grandparents are not on board with the Family Fit Plan, they could undo much of the progress that you've made with the kids and their habits around food, sleep, activity, screen time, and stress management. This is especially true if they live nearby and spend a lot of time helping you care for the kids.

Just as you helped your immediate family come on board, help your parents, in-laws, and other important family members come on board by sharing with them why you are doing the Family Fit Plan. Ask them if they would help you in reaching some of your family's goals. In fact, you might even consider inviting them to join you. Inviting them to come along with you, rather than dictating to them what to do, will make it more likely that they will support your changes, even if they don't agree with them. When they do something that shows they are trying, notice it and thank them. For example, if Grandma takes the kids to play at the park, you might thank her with a framed photograph of the kids swinging, riding a bike, or playing on the playground equipment. If Grandpa decides to take the kids to buy healthy sandwiches rather than fast food for lunch or dinner, commend him for such a healthy lunch idea and consider buying him a gift card for the sandwich shop so he can take the kids back again. If your mother-in-law goes outside her comfort zone to prepare a healthy dinner, take the extra effort to help the kids write a note to thank her for such a wonderful meal.

You can also make it a little easier on grandparents as they try to honor your requests by offering suggestions for meals, snacks, and activities based on your child's age and stage. For example, you might encourage your parents to take the baby for walks, read together, and play music. These are interactive activities that stimulate a child's rapidly growing brain. Although grandparents may be tempted to give in to a toddler's constant requests for the same not-so-healthy foods, you could share recipes and ideas to help them experiment with toddler favorites to make them a little bit healthier. (Check out the Smiling Faces Whole Wheat Pita Pizza, Baked Honey Mustard Chicken Fingers, and Whole Wheat Spinach Macaroni and Cheese in the Appendix for some ideas.)

As toddlers become preschoolers, they're more interested in trying new foods and activities. A great complement to a preschooler's high energy and short attention span are short adventures, such as taking the dog for a walk or going to the park or playground. A school-aged child is inquisitive and interested in trying out new experiences. A venture to a museum or aquarium, or a long hike in a local preserve or state or national forest, offers an opportunity for grandparent–grandchild bonding as well as ample opportunities for physical activity, conversation, and intellectual stimulation. A school-aged child also may be excited to learn to cook healthy and delicious foods with a grandparent. Perhaps a grandparent and teen could go on a trip to a state or national park, swim laps at the rec center, learn to lift weights together, or take a cooking class.

Co-parents

When the kids share time between homes, they are subject to the rules and habits in 2 homes of parents who love them but may approach how to raise them quite differently. It helps to get a sense of where other important influencers in your child's life stand on your journey to raise more fit and healthy kids. Although it is nice if your child's other parent agrees with your approach, ultimately, it's best to spend energy where you have control and to let be those areas where you do not have control. Kids are very place specific and can learn that different homes have different rules. You set the rules at your house, but other adults set their own rules at their house. As your kids come to adopt (and, hopefully, even enjoy) the changes that you've made, you can also help them to make better choices on their own and ask for changes that will make it more likely that they will achieve their goals.

School and Friends

Kids spend a lot of time at school, whether it be preschool, elementary, middle, or high school. The school culture and a child's peer network can have a big effect on a child's nutrition, physical activity, stress, screen time use, and even sleep. While parents continue to be highly influential throughout a child's life, as a child gets older the degree of parental influence lessens while school and peer influence increases. The methods you used to tell a child what to do or to eat work less well as a child increasingly spends more time outside the home away from parents. As kids age, parents lose a bit of control while kids gain it. For this reason, it helps to empower your kids to learn how to make good choices so that they make them even when you are not there. It also helps to advocate for a healthy school environment that supports good nutrition and activity, helps kids learn how to manage stressors, enforces responsible screen usage, and respects a child's need for adequate quality sleep. Figure 1.6 highlights common ways the school environment influences each of these factors.

Figure 1.6. School-Based Support Opportunities

	Before School	During School	After School
Nutrition	School breakfast, where applicable	School lunch Nutrition education	After-school programs: snacks After-school clubs: gardening, cooking
Physical activity	Walk/bike to school Running club	Physical education Recess Physical activity breaks	Sports programs Activity in after-school programs/child watch
Stress	Morning routines	Routines, learning, and peer interactions	Homework
Sleep	Start times	Naps in preschool	Homework
Screen usage	Morning routine	Digital curriculum School screen and smartphone policies	Homework Screen policies in after-school programs

You can't change everything, and you may not have enough time or energy during the day for it even if you could; however, as a parent you're ideally positioned to become a voice of change. Here are some examples of actions parents can take to help improve their children's health while they are in the school community.

- Attend school board and parent-teacher association meetings to advocate for increased time and resources for recess and physical education courses and healthier food choices in district schools.
- Join organizations such as Action for Healthy Kids (www.actionforhealthykids.org) or Alliance for a Healthier Generation (https://www.healthiergeneration.org), which are national initiatives with the goal of improving nutrition and physical education in schools.
- Join a school health advisory committee. These committees advise school administrators and the school board on various health-related topics, including overall health, physical activity, nutrition, tobacco prevention, and sex education. Committee members make recommendations regarding the number of hours in the school day that should be devoted to health and physical education and appropriate changes to improve the nutritional quality of foods offered in the school. As an active committee member, you would be well positioned to make change happen.
- Start a walking school bus in your neighborhood. Check out http://www.walkingschoolbus. org for a step-by-step guide to get started.

- Talk with your child's teacher and suggest ways to reward good behavior without using food incentives. Help to plan parties with healthy, delicious foods rather than pizza and ice cream.
- Encourage your school district to adopt and comply with the healthier school lunch standards.
- Support a school garden and nutrition education lessons.
- Ask your child's teacher if he or she would consider adding physical activity breaks into the day.
- Volunteer to lead a before- or after-school running club or recruit other parents or teachers who show interest.
- Become familiar with your school's electronic media policies and encourage responsible and limited use.
- Support efforts that advocate for delayed school start time for middle and high school students to increase their sleep time and positively affect their learning and general well-being.

For better or worse, your child's friends affect your child's health behaviors. In addition to learning more about the peers your child most admires, you can help nurture these friendships to improve your child's health. When it comes to physical activity, friends can influence each other to try new activities or sports that a child might otherwise resist. Additionally, peers are powerful models for trying new foods. By taking advantage of a child's sense of playful competition, activities such as the blindfold taste test described in week 2 could be a fun way to spend a Saturday afternoon. In fact, I have seen this play out through a community-based program I lead each week in which children and families meet with me at a park, where we walk together and then do a nutrition skill-building lesson. During one of those lessons, called "adventure," we help the kids be open to trying new things. We bring interesting fruits and vegetables like jicama, mango with chili lime powder, spicy edamame, and Asian pears. While few of the kids would willingly try some of those foods at the prompting of a parent, when done as a part of a taste test with peers, nearly everyone is willing to try everything.

Neighbors and Community

Your neighborhood and community can play an important role in helping you stick with your change plan. Individuals who feel emotional connectedness and a sense of belonging in their community experience improved health, according to research summarized by the Robert Wood Johnson Foundation. Among those surveyed, about half of adults feel a strong or moderate sense of membership in their communities, with just over 60% feeling a strong or moderate emotional connection. Figure 1.7 contains comments that are used to gauge your sense of community and help determine where you fit in your community with your sense of belonging and emotional connection and how you think this may affect your family's health.

Figure 1.7. How Connected Are You to Your Community?

Answer the following questions as they relate to the community where you currently live. The more "mostly" and "completely" answers, the more connected you are to your community.

	Not at all	Somewhat	Mostly	Completely
I can trust people in this community.				
I can recognize most of the members of this community.				
Most community members know me.				
This community has symbols and expressions of membership such as clothes, signs, art, architecture, logos, landmarks, and flags that people can recognize.				
I put a lot of time and effort into being part of this community.				
Being a member of this community is a part of my identity.				
It is very important to me to be a part of this community.				
I am with other community members a lot and enjoy being with them.				
I expect to be a part of this community for a long time.				
Members of this community have shared important events together, such as holidays, celebrations, or disasters.				
I feel hopeful about the future of this community.				
Members of this community care about each other.				
My community can work together to improve its health.				
My community has the resources to improve its health.				
My community works together to make positive change for health.				
I know my neighbors will help me stay healthy.				

Source: Adapted with permission from RAND. Well Being 425—Culture of Health.
https://alpdata.rand.org/index.php?page=data&p=showsurvey&syid=425. Accessed July 1, 2019.

If you want to improve the nutrition and fitness environment for children in your community, start by exploring your community's strengths and needs. What's already underway? What school and community policies interfere with supporting optimal nutrition and opportunities for activity?

Work and Colleagues

Working adults spend about half (or more) of their waking hours at work. Having a healthy work environment is important to sustain your changes. If you are lucky, your workplace offers healthful nutrition options in vending machines and cafeterias, encourages walking meetings and physical activity breaks, and rewards and celebrates employees in ways that don't usually involve sugary foods. If it hasn't, and you find yourself in an environment that is mostly inactive with candy jars on most desks, desserts in the break room, and soda in the vending machines, you will want to plan ahead for how to cope with an environment that does not support your healthful changes. Consider if there is any opportunity to positively influence your environment for the better. Can you go for a walk around the neighborhood during your break? Is it feasible to bring your lunch rather than eat out most days? Can you set a personal policy of not eating at your desk to minimize snacking and support more mindful eating? Is a standing desk an option?

Your Social Networks and Online Resources

In addition to your everyday contacts, whether those be family, neighbors, colleagues, or school staff and students, you may find leaning on your broader network can help to further reinforce your changes. For example, posting on Instagram or Facebook can help garner social support and a sense of accountability.

Family Meeting: Success Through Family Buy-in and Social Support

As your family continues to get ready to start the Family Fit Plan, use this second family meeting to explore how building social support outside your immediate family will help you achieve your goals.

✔ Open the meeting by asking everyone who their most important or influential relationship is outside your immediate family. For younger kids, you might ask who their best friend is. Follow this by asking how that person could help (or hinder) keeping up the healthy changes you are trying to make.

✔ **Activity:** Choose one of the following activities to do during your family meeting:
- Make a list of 2 to 3 things that would help make school and work healthier places that can help support your family.
- Complete the "How Connected Are You to Your Community?" worksheet (see Figure 1.7).
- Make a list of questions you'd like to ask your child's pediatrician at the next visit about your child's nutrition, fitness, or overall health. Use the "Previsit Checklist" as a guide (see Figure 1.3).
- Brainstorm ways to help a grandparent, co-parent, or other adult important in your child's life become more supportive of your healthy changes.

✔ **Closing family activity:** Close the family meeting by summarizing what you learned so far and anything you or your family finds interesting.

The Starting Line

What is your family's starting line when it comes to nutrition, physical activity, sleep, screen time, and stress management? For some areas you may simply need the equivalent of a 1-mile fun run to achieve your vision, while in others, you might need to brace yourself for a marathon. For example, does your family already have a consistent sleep routine, waking up each morning refreshed and ready to go? If so, you might not need to make much change to your sleep habits. On the other hand, are mealtimes difficult with more meals eaten out than at home, with very few vegetables or fruits consumed in a typical day? In that case, you might choose to focus more of your efforts over the coming weeks on nutrition.

You probably already have a gut feeling of how close you and your family's routines are to the recommendations or your ideals. This section includes several activities and assessments that help you put your gut feeling into more objective measurements. You can use this starting-line information to help set your goals (see Chapter 3), which is the final step of preparation before you start your Family Fit Plan. You also can use these pre-plan data to compare the changes between now and the end of the 30-day plan.

Nutrition: How Does Your Family Actually Eat?

Want to get a sense of how closely you and your family follow the nutrition recommendations for good health? The gold standard approach to figuring out your nutrition baseline is completing a 3-day food log, involving 2 typical weekdays and 1 weekend day. It's a bit challenging to capture the complete dietary intake of kids and teens, who may take in more than half of their total daily calories at school or after-school programs or when out with friends. Estimate portion sizes using your hand (see the KITCHEN HACKS "A 'Handy' Guide to Estimating Portions" Box).

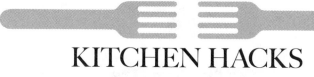

KITCHEN HACKS

A "Handy" Guide to Estimating Portions

Palm = 3 to 4 ounces. This is the recommended portion size for a piece of meat or fish.

Clenched fist = 1 cup. This is the recommended portion size for vegetables or fruits.

Front of a closed fist = ½ cup. This is the recommended portion size for whole grains and carbohydrates.

Cupped hand = 1 to 2 ounces. This is the recommended portion size for nuts or seeds.

Fingertip = 1 teaspoon. This is the recommended unit of measurement for butter.

Thumb = 2 tablespoons (or 1 ounce). This is the recommended portion size for peanut butter or cheese.

For practical purposes and for the Family Fit Plan, I recommend tracking and self-monitoring dietary intake through a written or photo food log. You can write down the time, type, and amount of all your food and drink intake for a day or use a free app such as MyFitnessPal or MealLogger. If you choose to do a photo log (my preference), you and any older kids who have a phone with a camera can quickly and easily take a snapshot of all of the food and drinks consumed each day the log is kept. For younger kids, you can take a photo of everything they eat or drink when they are with you, and then you can fill in the gaps by asking them (or an adult for the youngest kids) what they ate and drank at child care, preschool, school, and after-school programs or with the babysitter. You can review the photos or check the app to track intake. You don't need to do this every day, but the more you do it, the clearer picture you will get about you and your family's usual dietary intake.

Figure 2.1 shows a sample of one of my 1-day photo food logs. This was part of a week in which I tracked everything I ate or drank on my phone's camera roll—something I do every few months to keep tabs on my eating patterns and to note how close I am to achieving my daily recommendations.

Figure 2.1. My Daily Photo Food Log

Photo	Breakdown
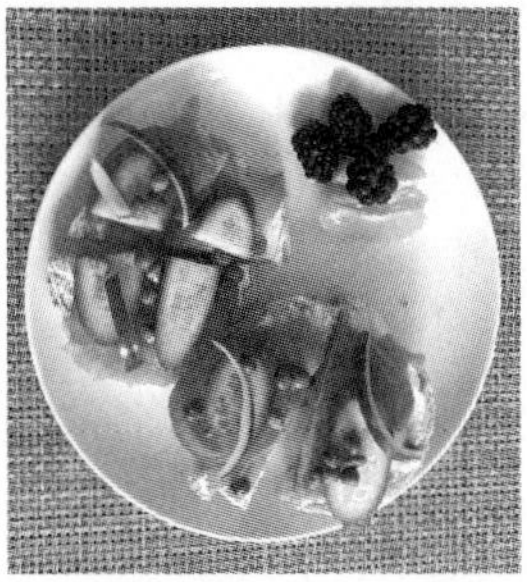	**Breakfast** 1 whole grain bagel (3 oz grain) 2 tablespoons cream cheese (other) 3 ounces smoked salmon (3 oz protein) ¼ cup tomatoes (¼ serving vegetables) ¼ cup cucumbers (¼ serving vegetables) ⅛ cup red onion (⅛ serving vegetables) 1 teaspoon capers (other) ½ mandarin orange (½ serving fruit) 4 blackberries (½ serving fruit)
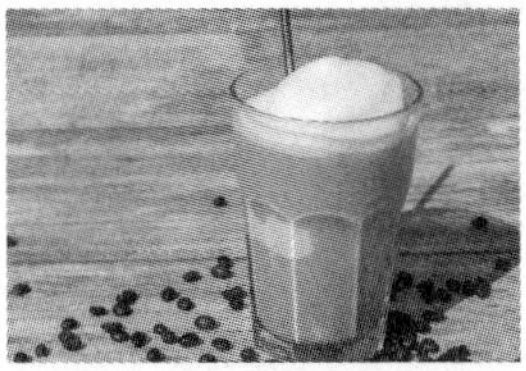	Unsweetened cold-brew iced coffee ¼ cup nonfat milk (¼ serving dairy)
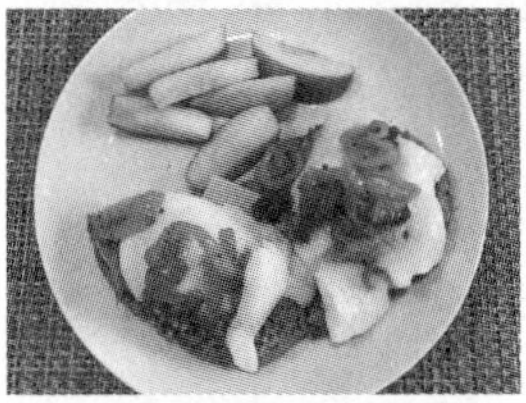	**Lunch** 2 slices whole grain bread (2 oz grain) 2 ounces cheddar cheese (2 servings dairy) 2 poached eggs (2 oz protein) ¼ cup marinated Italian peppers (¼ serving vegetable) 1 small apple (1 fruit)
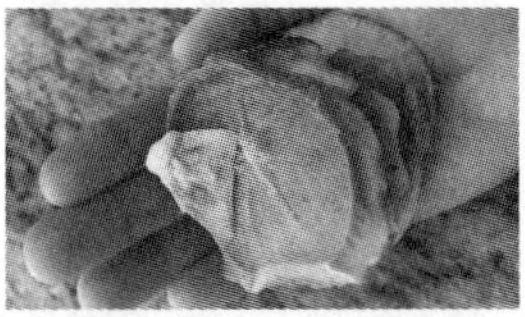	**Snack** ½ cup dried persimmons (1 fruit)
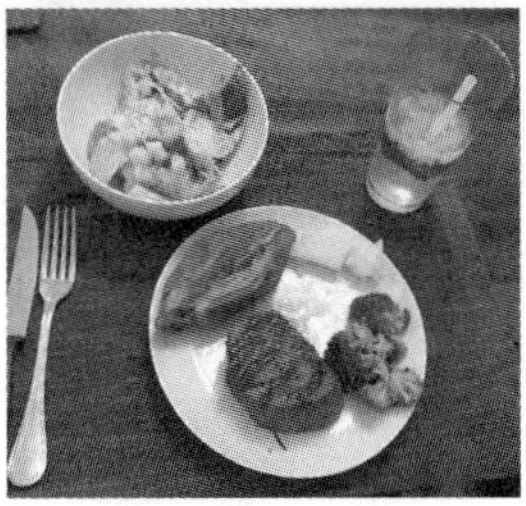	**Dinner** 4 ounces steak (4 oz protein) 1 medium sweet potato (1 serving vegetable) 1 tablespoon butter/cinnamon/honey (other) ½ cup roasted broccoli with a pinch of salt, ½ tsp olive oil (1 serving vegetable) ¼ cup pineapple (½ serving fruit) 1 cup Caesar salad including croutons, parmesan cheese, and romaine lettuce (1 serving vegetable) 1 tablespoon Caesar dressing (other) 1 sparkling water with lime and mint (other)
	Total: **Protein:** 9 ounce-equivalent **Grain:** 5 ounce-equivalent **Vegetables:** 3¾ cup-equivalent **Fruit:** 3½ cup-equivalent **Dairy:** 2¼ cup-equivalent

You'll notice that I summed the food groups (protein, grain, vegetables, fruits, and dairy) into ounce or cup-equivalents (quantity equivalents). For reference, quantity equivalents for each food group are:

- Vegetables and fruits, 1 cup-equivalent is 1 cup raw or cooked vegetable or fruit, 1 cup vegetable or fruit juice, 2 cups leafy salad greens, ½ cup dried fruit or vegetable.
- Grains, 1 ounce-equivalent is ½ cup cooked rice, pasta, or cereal; 1 ounce dry pasta or rice; 1 medium (1 ounce) slice of bread; 1 ounce of ready-to-eat cereal (about 1 cup of flaked cereal).
- Dairy, 1 cup-equivalent is 1 cup milk, yogurt, or fortified soymilk; 1½ ounces natural cheese such as cheddar cheese or 2 ounces of processed cheese.
- Protein foods, 1 ounce-equivalent is 1 ounce lean meat, poultry, or seafood; 1 egg; ¼ cup cooked beans or tofu; 1 Tbsp peanut butter; ½ ounce nuts or seeds.

What do you do with this information? Fill in Figure 2.2 to get a sense of what a typical day looks like for each family member. Help school-aged and older kids complete their own worksheet. (They can think of it as a "fun" hands-on way to practice some math. See Appendix.) The more engaged they are in each step of this process, the more likely they will be to feel ownership over their health and the changes being made, and the outcome will be much better. If you feel like tracking and calculating food intake seems like kind of a drag—you are not alone. It can feel quite tedious, but even if you only do this once or twice, it can give you a lot of insight into how your family typically eats.

Figure 2.2. Making Sense of Your Photo Food Log

Using your photo food log, complete the following worksheet for each day for each family member. Use the photos to estimate food amounts and leave a tally representing the amount eaten from each of the food groups. Figure 2.3 is an example of what my log looks like at the end of one day.

	Breakfast	Lunch	Dinner	Snack	Total
Fruit 1 cup-equiv of fruit is: • 1 cup of raw or cooked fruit • ½ cup of dried fruit • 1 cup of 100% fruit juice					(cups)
Vegetables 1 cup-equiv of vegetables is: • 1 cup of raw or cooked vegetables • 2 cups of leafy salad greens • 1 cup of 100% vegetable juice					(cups)
Protein 1 ounce-equiv of protein is: • 1 ounce of lean meat, poultry, or seafood • 1 egg • 1 tablespoon of peanut butter • ¼ cup of cooked beans or peas • ½ ounce of nuts or seeds					(ounces)
Grains 1 ounce-equiv of grains is: • 1 slice of bread • 1 ounce of ready-to-eat cereal • ½ cup of cooked rice, pasta, or cereal					(ounces)
Dairy/Substitute 1 cup-equiv of dairy is: • 1 cup of milk • 1 cup of yogurt • 1 cup of fortified soy beverage • 1½ ounces of natural cheese or 2 ounces of processed cheese					(cups)

Figure 2.3. Example: My 1-Day Food Log Worksheet

	Breakfast	Lunch	Dinner	Snack	Total
Fruit 1 cup-equiv of fruits is • 1 cup of raw or cooked fruit • ½ cup of dried fruit • 1 cup of 100% fruit juice	½ mandarin orange 4 blackberries	1 small apple (1 serving fruit)	¼ cup of pineapple (½ serving fruit)	½ cup of dried persimmons (1 serving fruit)	(cups) 3
Vegetables 1 cup-equiv of vegetables is • 1 cup of raw or cooked vegetables • 2 cups of leafy salad greens • 1 cup of 100% vegetable juice	¼ cup of tomatoes ¼ cup of cucumbers ⅛ cup of red onion	¼ cup of marinated Italian peppers (¼ serving vegetable)	1 medium sweet potato (1 serving vegetable) ½ cup of roasted broccoli w/salt, ½ teaspoon of olive oil (1 serving vegetable) 1 cup Caesar salad including croutons, Parmesan cheese, and romaine lettuce (1 serving vegetable)		(cups) 3¾
Protein 1 ounce-equiv protein is • 1 ounce of lean meat, poultry, or seafood • 1 egg • 1 tablespoon of peanut butter • ¼ cup of cooked beans or peas • ½ ounce of nuts or seeds	3 oz of smoked salmon	2 poached eggs (2 oz protein)	4 ounces of steak (4 oz protein)		(ounces) 9
Grains 1 ounce-equiv of grain is • 1 slice of bread • 1 ounce of ready-to-eat cereal • ½ cup of cooked rice, pasta, or cereal	1 whole grain bagel (3 oz grain)	2 slices of whole grain bread (2 oz grain)			(ounces) 5
Dairy/Substitute 1 cup-equiv of dairy is • 1 cup of milk • 1 cup of yogurt • 1 cup of fortified soy beverage • 1½ ounces of natural cheese or 2 ounces of processed cheese	¼ cup nonfat milk	2 ounces cheddar cheese (1 cup equivalent)			(cups) 1¼

You will refer back to these logs when you compare your actual intake with the recommendations and set goals (see Chapter 3).

Physical Activity: What's Your Current Activity Level?

An activity tracker can help you figure out your family's current activity level. Although adults have many options to choose from, there are fewer options for kids, whose activity can be somewhat difficult to track. You don't need an ultra-sophisticated device. Something as simple as a step counter pedometer is good enough to help you get a sense of the number of steps you and your kids take in a day. Or, estimate your kids' activity level by adding up how many minutes per day a child spends being active such as walking or biking to and from school, physical education class, active play at recess or during preschool or daycare, and sports or other activities after school. Track estimated activity using Figure 2.4 (and in the Appendix).

Figure 2.4. Keeping Tabs on Physical Activity
Record the types and minutes of activity for each family member for each day of the week. Put a ★ next to each day that a child was active for 60 minutes or more or an adult was active for 30 minutes or more. Use this format for all family members.

Family Member	Mon	Tues	Wed	Thurs	Fri	Sat	Sun

For kids, consider physical activity
- Before school (eg, walk or bike to school, running club)
- During school (eg, physical education class, recess)
- After school (eg, sports, walk or bike home)

For adults, consider physical activity
- During the workday (eg, walking meetings, a walk to get lunch or exercise during lunch or breaks)
- Before or after work (eg, devoted time to the gym or a sport)
- Before bed (eg, calisthenics, yoga)
- Recreational time (eg, sports, walks with friends, swimming)
- Housework (yard work, cleaning and vacuuming, etc)

Fitness Testing in Schools

Some school districts use fitness testing such as the FitnessGram, developed by the Cooper Institute in 1982 and used in thousands of schools across the United States. These assessments provide parents with a report of a child's fitness level based on standardized fitness tests to measure cardiovascular fitness, muscular strength and endurance, flexibility, and body mass index. In fact, my son's biggest motivation for our Family Fit Plan was to prepare for the 5th grade FitnessGram assessment at his school. If you really want to get a sense of where you're starting from, consider putting yourself (and any interested family members!) through a baseline fitness assessment, a modification of the FitnessGram, described in the GET FIT! "The Family Fitness Assessment" Box.

💪 GET FIT! THE FAMILY FITNESS ASSESSMENT

There are 5 components of fitness: cardiovascular fitness, muscular strength, muscular endurance, flexibility, and body composition. Many times, muscular strength and endurance are assessed together. The following is an optional group of assessments you can do before and after the first 4 weeks of using the *Family Fit Plan*. It will take you about 45 minutes if you complete all the assessments at one time. Results may be helpful in creating your SMART goals (see Chapter 3). It also may be helpful for you to see your progress when comparing your before and after fitness levels. Use the log in Figure 2.5 to track your overall fitness. Remember, this is just a baseline! Be sensitive when taking measurements and allow family members to decline assessments that they don't want to do.

1. **Cardiovascular fitness**
   One-mile walk/run. Go to your nearest track (a standard track is ¼ mile around), or treadmill, or calculate a 1-mile distance in your neighborhood. Complete the mile as quickly as you can. Record this time.

2. **Muscular strength and endurance**
   Check your abdominal strength and endurance with the abdominal crunch. Do as many as you can with good form in 2 minutes. Record this number.

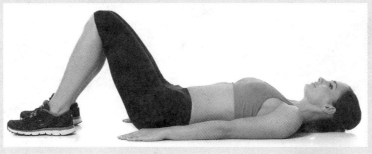

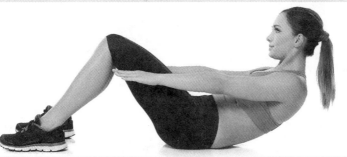

Abdominal crunch

When positioning yourself to do an abdominal crunch, be sure to engage the abdominal muscles and press your lower back toward the floor or mat prior to using your abdominal muscles to lift your back off the floor. Avoid using your arms to pull on your neck, back, or hips to lift your body.

(continued)

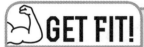 **GET FIT!** **THE FAMILY FITNESS ASSESSMENT** (*continued*)

Check your upper body strength and endurance with the push-up or modified push-up. Do as many as you can with good form either before you become fatigued or within 2 minutes. Record this number.

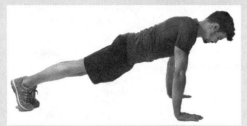 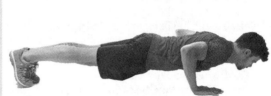

Push-up

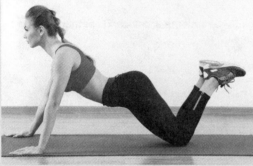 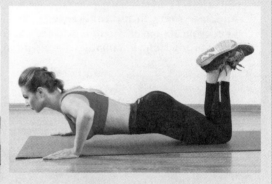

Modified push-up

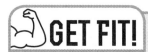 **GET FIT!** **THE FAMILY FITNESS ASSESSMENT** (*continued*)

3. **Flexibility**
   Measure your shoulder flexibility with the shoulder stretch test. Note whether your fingers touch, or, if not, have a family member use a ruler to measure the distance between them. Record this distance.

4. **Body composition**
   The preferred methods to assess body composition includes estimation of lean muscle mass with tools such as skinfold measurements or bioelectrical impedance analysis. These are not readily available tools for home use. For a general approximation, we will use body mass index and waist circumference measurements. Body mass index is a measure of height and weight. Record each family member's height and weight. Then enter that data along with the demographic information requested in the Centers for Disease Control and Prevention body mass index calculator for adults or children, both available at http://cdc.gov/BMI.

   Waist circumference is measured by using a measuring tape to measure the narrowest part of the waist.

   To correctly measure waist circumference

   • Stand and place a tape measure around your middle, just above your hip bones.
   • Make sure tape is horizontal around the waist.
   • Keep the tape snug around the waist but not compressing the skin.
   • Measure your waist just after you breathe out.

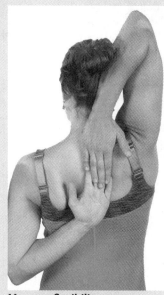

Measure flexibility

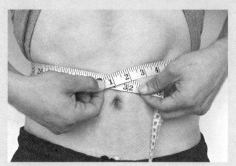

Waist circumference

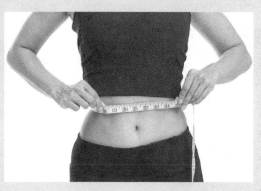

Figure 2.5. Fitness Assessment Log

Date:

Family Member	1 Mile Time	Crunches (total in 2 min)	Push-ups/ Modified Push-ups (total in 2 min)	Shoulder Stretch Distance Right (R) Left (L)	Waist Circumference (inches)	Height (ft, in)	Weight (lb)	BMI (number for adult or % for child/ adolescent)[a]

Abbreviation: BMI, body mass index.

[a] BMI is height (in meters)/weight (in kg). Use the Centers for Disease Control and Prevention BMI calculator to determine BMI for adults and BMI percentiles for children and teens (http://cdc.gov/BMI).

Sleep: Your Family's Starting Point

While many activity trackers will also assess your sleep duration and quality, an easy and low-tech way to track sleep is to keep a paper and pencil log of it. Over the course of the next week, use the sleep log from the National Sleep Foundation (Figure 2.6 and Appendix) for yourself and the kids' sleep log for your young kids. Older kids should complete their own log.

Figure 2.6. Sleep Logs
Adults Tracker
Track your family's sleep behaviors using these sleep logs.

🦫 N A T I O N A L S L E E P F O U N D A T I O N

SLEEP LOG: Please fill this out for the previous day and night no more than 3 hours after waking. The information can be an estimate when necessary. This sleep log is provided by the National Sleep Foundation, www.sleepfoundation.org.

NAME _____   WEEK OF _____

DAY	Sun	Mon	Tues	Wed	Thurs	Fri	Sat
1. Did you nap? a. For how long? b. At what time?	Yes No ____min	Yes No ____min	Yes No ____min	Yes No ____min	Yes No ____min	Yes No ____min	Yes No ____min
2. Did you have any caffeine* after 6pm?	Yes No	Yes No	Yes No	Yes No	Yes No	Yes No	Yes No
3. Did you drink alcohol after 6pm?	Yes No	Yes No	Yes No	Yes No	Yes No	Yes No	Yes No
4. Did you use nicotine after 6pm?	Yes No	Yes No	Yes No	Yes No	Yes No	Yes No	Yes No
5. Did you exercise?	Yes No	Yes No	Yes No	Yes No	Yes No	Yes No	Yes No
6. Did you eat a heavy meal or snack after 6pm?	Yes No	Yes No	Yes No	Yes No	Yes No	Yes No	Yes No
7. Did you take any sleeping medication a. What medication? b. Amount c. At what time?	Yes No ____ ____ ____	Yes No ____ ____ ____	Yes No ____ ____ ____	Yes No ____ ____ ____	Yes No ____ ____ ____	Yes No ____ ____ ____	Yes No ____ ____ ____
8. Were you sleepy during the day?	Yes No	Yes No	Yes No	Yes No	Yes No	Yes No	Yes No
NIGHT							
1. What time did you turn off the lights to go to sleep?							
2. What time did you wake up?							
3. How many total hours did you sleep?							
4. How many times did you wake up in the night?							
5. Rate the quality of your sleep: 1=poor, 5=excellent							
6. Do you feel you got enough sleep?							

Caffeine = coffee, tea, caffeinated soda, chocolate, energy drinks, certain medications.

Reprinted with permission from https://sleepfoundation.org/sites/default/files/
sample_sleep_log-by_national_sleep_foundation.pdf

(continued)

Figure 2.6. Sleep Logs *(continued)*
Kids Tracker

Day	Sun	Mon	Tues	Wed	Thurs	Fri	Sat
How was your child's mood and energy during the day? (good, OK, bad)							
How well did your child pay attention at school or home? (not at all, OK, great)							
Did your child take a nap? If yes, when and for how long?							
Did your child consume any caffeine (eg, soda, chocolate, tea)? If yes, at what time?							
Did your child exercise? If yes, when and for how long?							
Did your child use a screen (eg, TV, tablet, phone) within 1 hour of bedtime?							
Did your child follow a bedtime routine? If yes, what?							
Night	**Sun**	**Mon**	**Tues**	**Wed**	**Thurs**	**Fri**	**Sat**
What time did your child go to bed?							
How easily did your child fall asleep?							
How many times did your child wake in the night?							
How many total hours did your child sleep?							
Was your child disturbed by any noise, lights, temperature, sound, nightmares, stress, pain, hunger, thirst, etc? If so, by what?							
When your child woke for the day, was s/he well rested?							

Adapted with permission from http://www.sleepforkids.org/pdf/SleepDiary.pdf

Look back at the week. Do you notice any patterns—for better or for worse? You can use this information to help you in setting sleep goals in Chapter 3.

Screen Time: Your Family's Starting Point

You can use any of a number of apps and phone and electronic device settings to track screen time use. Some examples include Moment, unGlue Kids, Bosco, Bark, and Circle by Disney. Or you can use the American Academy of Pediatrics (AAP) Media Time Calculator, available at www.healthychildren.org/mediauseplan, to get a sense of how much of your child's day is spent using screens.

Stress: Your Family's Starting Point

How much stress are your family members under? How do they handle the stress? To figure out your family's starting point, have a conversation about stress. Ask open-ended questions such as, "What is on your mind?" While young kids may not be able to tell you that they are feeling stress, some body signs of stress can help clue you in. Although any of the following signs may occur for other reasons, if you notice an ongoing change in any of them, consider stress as a possible contributing factor. If the signs continue, talk to your child's pediatrician.

- **Physical signs:** constantly tired; difficulty sleeping; change in eating routines; frequently sick; increased headaches, body aches, and pain; stomach pain, constipation, or diarrhea
- **Behavioral signs:** difficulty concentrating; difficulty remembering; laughing or crying for no reason; increased anger or tantrums; physical aggression; feeling anxious; decreased enjoyment of usual activities; withdrawing from social situations; relationship problems; restlessness

In addition to getting a sense of how much stress your family is experiencing, it helps to identify ways that different family members cope with stress. Figure 2.7 can help you identify some ways that you or other adults cope with stress. Some ways of coping are more productive; others may be more detrimental. One of thegoals of the Family Fit Plan is to help your family cope with stress in ways that are most productive.

Figure 2.7. How Do You Cope With Stress?

Review the following statements, which include ways that people often cope with stressors. Think about how you normally cope with stressful situations. Check if you do or do not use the particular coping strategy. Make your answers as true for you as you can.

Example	I do this a lot.	I do not do this a lot.	Type of Coping
I do something to think about it less, such as going to movies, watching TV, reading, daydreaming, sleeping, shopping [or exercising].			Self-distraction (A)
I take action to try to make the situation better.			Active coping (A)
I say to myself, "This isn't real."			Denial (M)
I use alcohol or other drugs [or food] to make myself feel better.			Substance use (M)
I get emotional support from others.			Use of emotional support (A)
I get help and advice from other people.			Instrumental support (A)
I give up the attempt to cope.			Behavioral disengagement (M)
I say things to let my unpleasant feelings escape.			Venting (M)
I look for something good in what is happening.			Positive reframing (A)
I try to come up with a strategy about what to do.			Planning (A)
I make jokes about it.			Humor (A)
I accept the reality of the fact that it has happened.			Acceptance (A)
I pray or meditate.			Religion/spirituality (A)
I blame myself for things that happened.			Self-blame (M)

Abbreviations: A, adaptive, or generally helpful coping strategy; M, maladaptive, or generally unhelpful coping strategy.

Adapted with permission from Springer Nature Customer Service Centre GmbH: Springer Nature.

Carver CS. You want to measure coping but your protocol's too long: consider the brief COPE. *Int J Behav Med*. 1997;4(1):92–100

Family Meeting: The Starting Line

The focus of the third family meeting is determining the family starting line for each of the 5 health behaviors: nutrition, physical activity, sleep, screen time, and stress.

✔ Open the meeting by asking family members to share separately what they already do that they think makes them healthy.

✔ Share with your family that the purpose of the meeting is to find out what your family members' usual habits are in the 5 health behaviors. The starting point is just that— a starting point. Encourage everyone to be completely honest in answering the questions. You aren't aiming for any particular goal yet. You just want to learn your starting point. Whatever it is, it is OK.

✔ **Activity:** Complete Figure 2.7 to figure out how you and your family members cope with stress. Discuss this together.

✔ **Activity:** The AAP Media Time Calculator. Use the AAP Media Time Calculator (www.healthychildren.org/mediauseplan) for each child to approximate how much time in a typical day he or she spends in out-of-school screen time activities. You might be shocked (especially for teens!).

✔ **Activity for the week:** Schedule the other baseline activities. Together, come up with a plan for when you will complete some or all of the following activities:

- **A 3-day food log.** Ideally include 2 weekdays and 1 weekend day. Come up with a plan for what type of tracking method you will use. If you use a written or photo food log, track your intake by food group using Figure 2.2.
- **The baseline physical activity log.** Decide on what method of tracking you would like to use, whether it is completing the form (see Figure 2.5) or using a pedometer or an activity tracker.
- **The 1-week sleep log and follow-up questions.** Older kids and adults should complete the form in Figure 2.6 themselves, but parents will need to complete the form for younger children.
- **The baseline fitness assessment.** Carve out about 45 minutes in your weekend or other convenient day and time to complete some or all of the baseline fitness assessments described in the GET FIT! "The Family Fitness Assessment" Box.

✔ **Closing family activity:** Close with a question. What did you learn about your health habits from these activities? What do you expect to find out when we do the other assessments?

On Your Mark...Get Set...Goal!

The final step of your planning is setting goals and a schedule to create new habits and routines that will bring your Family Fit Plan to life and help you and your family achieve your vision of optimal family health and fitness.

Goal Setting

Goal setting is a bit of an art. Goals are more likely to be met if they are SMART goals, which are goals that are *s*pecific, *m*easurable, *a*ttainable, *r*elevant, and *t*ime bound.

You are likely to be more successful if you focus on creating *positive goals* that do more of something (eg, eat vegetables, drink water), rather than goals that avoid or prevent something (eg, stop eating dessert, prevent diabetes). In addition, aim for *mastery goals,* which focus on learning new skills (eg, learning to cook), rather than performance goals, which focus on achieving a particular outcome (eg, weight loss). For example, instead of the goal, "We would like to eat healthier," a SMART, positive, mastery goal would be, "We will eat healthier by eating at least 5 vegetables and fruits per day for the next 30 days." Next, list 2 or 3 action steps you will take to achieve each goal. For example, if 1 of your SMART goals is "to eat at least 5 vegetables and fruits per day for the next 30 days," your action steps might be as follows:

❶ I will go grocery shopping at least 1 time per week so that we always have fruits and vegetables in the house.

❷ I will include a salad with each dinner so that we are guaranteed to have a minimum of 2 vegetables available.

❸ I will make sure to eat a fruit with breakfast every day.

Refer to the Family Fit Plan (Figure 3.1) for some sample goals; feel free to use these or create your own. Note that some of the actions included in the sample plan have not been discussed yet. Don't worry; they will be as we dive into the 4 weeks of the Family Fit Plan soon.

The results of your baseline assessments of nutrition, physical activity, sleep, screen time, and stress can be useful in helping you set goals for the month ahead. Of course, you don't need to make changes in all 5 areas at once. In fact, you may be most successful if you focus on one area at a time. As you reach your goal in 1 area, you can set new goals in that area or start another goal in 1 of the other 5 areas. In other words, tailor the Family Fit Plan to your family's needs and vision. My family ended up doing the Family Fit Plan a few times, focusing on goals in different areas each time. Set goals that feel most important, relevant, and doable for your family.

Figure 3.1. The Family Fit Plan

This is a sample Family Fit Plan that lists specific, measurable, attainable, relevant, and time-bound (SMART) goals and actions.

THE SAMPLE FAMILY FIT PLAN			
Our "Why": To be a stronger, healthier, and happier family			
Our Vision: By the end of the 30 days, the "recommended" nutrition, activity, sleep, screen, and stress behaviors will be a usual part of our everyday routines and habits.			

	SMART Goal 1	Action 1	Action 2	Action 3
Nutrition	Eat 5 vegetables and fruits per day.	Offer a fruit and/ or vegetable at each meal and snack.	Go grocery shopping at least once per week, and buy a variety of vegetables and fruits.	Keep a filled bowl of fruit on the kitchen counter.
	SMART Goal 2	**Action 1**	**Action 2**	**Action 3**
	Eat family dinner together at least 3 days per week.	Build a set dinnertime into the schedule each night.	Make a weekly meal plan.	Learn to cook easy and fast family meals.
	SMART Goal 3	**Action 1**	**Action 2**	**Action 3**
	Drink water or milk only, most of the time.	Purchase only milk and regular or sparkling water at the store.	Fill a water bottle for each family member each morning.	Purchase a fruit infuser pitcher to improve the taste of the water.
Physical activity	**SMART Goal 1**	**Action 1**	**Action 2**	**Action 3**
	Get at least 30 minutes of physical activity every day for adults and 60 minutes for kids.	Walk for 15 minutes after dinner most nights.	Walk or bike to work, school, restaurant, etc at least 1 time per week.	Train for a 5K or other fun event to complete in the next 1 to 2 months.
	SMART Goal 2	**Action 1**	**Action 2**	**Action 3**
	Do muscle strengthening exercise at least 2 days per week.	Complete the 7-minute workout at least 2 days per week.	Do crunches and push-ups for 30 seconds before bed each night.	Play on the playground, including the monkey bars, with the kids, 1 time per week.
	SMART Goal 3	**Action 1**	**Action 2**	**Action 3**
	Be active together as a family at least 1 time per week.	Choose a family fitness activity to do together each Sunday.	Invite the whole family to go for a walk together after dinner.	Include a brief physical activity in family meetings.

	SMART Goal	Action 1	Action 2	Action 3
Sleep	Sleep for the recommended number of hours per night.	Go to bed at the same time each night.	Follow the 5Bs bedtime routine: Bath Brush Book Breathe Bed	Remove screens (TV, phones, computers, tablets) from the bedroom.
	SMART Goal	**Action 1**	**Action 2**	**Action 3**
Screen time	Spend 2 hours or less on nonwork and nonschool screen time per day.	Develop a schedule for screen time. Avoid screen time within 1 hour of bedtime.	Implement a screen-free policy for mealtimes and snack times.	Remove screens from bedrooms.
	SMART Goal	**Action 1**	**Action 2**	**Action 3**
Stress management	Each family member will learn and practice 2 to 3 new ways to manage stress and anxiety.	Learn how to meditate, and practice meditating for at least 10 minutes 3 times per week.	Learn and practice mindful breathing at least 3 times per week.	Practice the STOP mindfulness activity each time a stressful experience occurs over the next 4 weeks: Stop what you are doing. Take a deep breath. Observe what is happening. Proceed.

Nutrition: What and How We Should Eat

Every year, the US government publishes a document called the Dietary Guidelines for Americans. The Dietary Guidelines include recommendations for how to eat to optimize health. While the report is generally hundreds of pages long, the most recent guidelines can be boiled down to a simple visual called MyPlate. It applies to every age group and can be easily modified for family members who have food allergies or other restrictions (Figure 3.2).

Figure 3.2. MyPlate

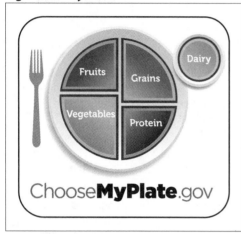

Source: https://choosemyplate.gov

Think of MyPlate as showing 6 key messages. Keeping these messages in mind while you choose and prepare foods can help your whole family eat better with little fuss.

Message 1: Think of foods in terms of food groups.

MyPlate includes 5 food groups—vegetables, fruits, (whole) grains, protein, and dairy. Although some foods can fit into more than 1 group—for example, black beans can be considered a protein and a vegetable—most foods generally fall into 1 category. As you are planning meals, packing lunches, eating out, or putting together snacks, keep the food groups in mind. Try to choose vegetables and fruits that are brightly colored. Go for grains that are whole grains (eg, whole wheat bread, brown rice, oatmeal, and quinoa, as opposed to white bread, white rice, and white cereals). Whole-grain foods have more fiber and are more likely to contribute to feelings of fullness. Pick proteins that are healthier (eg, seafood, nuts and seeds, poultry, eggs) and minimize how often you eat red or processed meats. If you eat red meat, choose round or loin for the leanest cuts. Try to include a dairy product or dairy substitute 2 or 3 times per day to make sure you get enough calcium and vitamin D for strong bones. Figure 3.3 lists MyPlate food group recommendations for the family by age, gender, and activity level. Compare your nutrition intake from your food log (see Chapter 2) to the MyPlate recommendations. How close are your eating patterns to the recommendations? In what food groups do you eat more or less than recommended? If you're like most people, you probably get more than enough grains and proteins and too few vegetables and fruits.

Figure 3.3. How Much of What Should We Eat?

Use this table to estimate your and your family's daily nutritional needs.[a]

	1–3 years	4–8 years	9–13 years	14–18 years	19–40 years	41–60 years	61+ years
Calories							
Female	900–1,000	1,200	1,400–1,600	1,800	1,800–2,000	1,800	1,600
Male	900–1,200	1,200–1,400	1,600–2,000	2,000–2,400	2,400	2,200	2,000
Milk/dairy	2 cups	2½ cups	3 cups	3 cups	3 cups	3 cups	3 cups
Lean meat/ fish/beans/ nuts/eggs							
Female	2 ounces	3 ounces	5 ounces	5 ounces	5 ounces	5 ounces	5 ounces
Male	3 ounces	4 ounces	6 ounces	6 ounces	6½ ounces	6 ounces	5½ ounces
Fruits							
Female	1 cup	1½ cups	1½ cups	1½ cups	1½–2 cups	1½ cups	1½ cups
Male	1 cup	1½ cups	1½ cups	2 cups	2 cups	2 cups	2 cups
Vegetables							
Female	1 cup	1½ cups	2 cups	2½ cups	2½ cups	2½ cups	2 cups
Male	1½ cups	1½ cups	2½ cups	3 cups	3 cups	3 cups	2½ cups
Grains							
Female	3 ounces	4 ounces	5 ounces	6 ounces	6 ounces	6 ounces	5 ounces
Male	3 ounces	5 ounces	6 ounces	7 ounces	8 ounces	7 ounces	6 ounces
"Extra" calories[b]							
Female	150	100	120	170	210	170	130
Male	150	100	200	300	350	280	270

[a] Estimated calorie needs are based on a sedentary lifestyle. Kids and adults who are physically active have higher calories needs of about 0 to 200 kcal/day for people who are moderately active and 200 to 400 kcal/day for people who are very physically active. *Sedentary* means a lifestyle that includes only the physical activity of daily living. *Moderately active* means a lifestyle that, in addition to the activities of daily living, includes an equivalent to walking about 1½ to 3 miles per day at a brisk pace. *Very physically active* means a lifestyle that includes an equivalent to walking more than 3 miles per day at a brisk pace. Estimates for women do not include women who are pregnant or breastfeeding.

[b] Extra calories include calories from additional servings of the food groups or added oils or sugars. As a general rule, aim for calories from sweets, desserts, sugary drinks, and other "extra" foods consumed to add up to no more than the amount of extra calories noted in the box.

Source: Adapted from https://health.gov/dietaryguidelines/2015/guidelines/appendix-3 and https://health.gov/dietaryguidelines/2015/guidelines/appendix-2.

Foods in each group include

✔ **Vegetables**

- Dark-green vegetables: All fresh, frozen, and canned dark-green leafy vegetables and broccoli, cooked or raw (eg, broccoli; spinach; romaine; kale; collard, turnip, and mustard greens).
- Red and orange vegetables: All fresh, frozen, and canned red and orange vegetables or juice, cooked or raw (eg, tomatoes, tomato juice, red peppers, carrots, sweet potatoes, winter squash, pumpkin).
- Legumes (beans and peas): All cooked from dry or canned beans and peas (eg, kidney beans, white beans, black beans, lentils, chickpeas, pinto beans, split peas, edamame [green soybeans]). Does not include green beans or green peas.
- Starchy vegetables: All fresh, frozen, and canned starchy vegetables (eg, white potatoes, corn, green peas, green lima beans, plantains, cassava).
- Other vegetables: All other fresh, frozen, and canned vegetables, cooked or raw (eg, iceberg lettuce, green beans, onions, cucumbers, cabbage, celery, zucchini, mushrooms, green peppers).

✔ **Fruits**

- All fresh, frozen, canned, and dried fruits and fruit juices (eg, oranges and orange juice, apples and apple juice, bananas, grapes, melons, berries, raisins). Note: aim to get all fruit servings from fruit rather than fruit juice.

✔ **Grains**

- Whole grains: All whole-grain products and whole grains used as ingredients (eg, whole wheat bread, whole-grain cereals and crackers, oatmeal, quinoa, popcorn, brown rice).
- Refined grains: All refined-grain products and refined grains used as ingredients (eg, white breads, refined grain cereals and crackers, pasta, white rice). Refined grain choices should be enriched.

✔ **Dairy**

- All milk, including lactose-free and lactose-reduced products and fortified soy beverages (soy milk), yogurt, frozen yogurt, dairy desserts, and cheeses. Most choices should be fat-free or low-fat. Cream, sour cream, and cream cheese are not included due to their low calcium content.

✔ **Protein foods**

- All seafood, meats, poultry, eggs, soy products, nuts, and seeds. Meats and poultry should be lean or low-fat, and nuts should be unsalted. Legumes (beans and peas) can be considered part of this group as well as the vegetable group, but they should be counted in 1 group only.

Quantity equivalents for each food group are

- Vegetables and fruits, 1 cup-equivalent is 1 cup of raw or cooked vegetable or fruit, 1 cup of vegetable or fruit juice, 2 cups of leafy salad greens, and ½ cup of dried fruit or vegetable.
- Grains, 1 ounce-equivalent is ½ cup of cooked rice, pasta, or cereal; 1 ounce dry pasta or rice; 1 medium (1 ounce) slice of bread; and 1 ounce of ready-to-eat cereal (about 1 cup of flaked cereal).
- Dairy, 1 cup-equivalent is 1 cup of milk, yogurt, or fortified soy milk, and 1½ ounces of natural cheese such as cheddar cheese or 2 ounces of processed cheese.
- Protein foods, 1 ounce-equivalent is 1 ounce of lean meat, poultry, or seafood; 1 egg; ¼ cup of cooked beans or tofu; 1 tablespoon of peanut butter; and ½ ounce of nuts or seeds.

Source: Adapted from the Dietary Guidelines for Americans https://health.gov/dietaryguidelines/2015/guidelines/appendix-3/

Message 2: "Balanced" does not mean equal.

Note that the plate is half filled with vegetables and fruits. This is the target when choosing and preparing meals. Try to include at least 2 vegetables or 1 fruit and 1 vegetable with meals. Generally, most people eat a lot more protein and grains than they need and far fewer fruits and vegetables. A balanced eating plan is high in vegetables and fruits and moderate in grains and protein. The best grains are whole grains rather than heavily processed "white" grains.

Message 3: Choose meals over snacks.

The plate represents a balanced meal and is a good reminder that most of the food we eat should be eaten during mealtimes. Most kids and many adults get far more calories from snacks and drinks than is recommended. Aim for 3 balanced meals during the day and snacks (mostly fruits and vegetables) at prescheduled times. Offer kids water to drink between meals and water or milk at meals.

Message 4: Sit down at a table to eat.

A visual of a plate is a good reminder that it is best if we eat food sitting down at a table and using a plate, rather than eating on the run or in front of the computer, smartphone, television, or other electronic device.

Message 5: Notice what's missing.

You may have noticed that the plate does not include any sugary foods or drinks or added fats, such as butter and oil. It's not that you should never eat these foods, but try to avoid including them with meals most of the time. What tends to work the best is if you plan for dessert days—for example, on Mondays and Thursdays. That way, the family can occasionally have the less healthy foods that they like, and you can head off some of the begging, pleading, nagging, or expectation for dessert after every dinner. Limit sugary drinks to no more than 8 ounces (1 cup) per week, ideally less. The MyPlate meal plans include an "extra calories" allot-ment. This is where desserts and added fats or extra amounts from the food groups fit in. The idea is that if people stay within their calorie range overall, they will likely maintain a healthy weight. It is not necessary to count calories most of the time, although you might want to notice how many calories are in junk foods like candy bars and sodas, because the extra calo-ries can add up quickly, either from extra amounts of some of the food groups or added fats and sugars.

Message 6: Go small.

Although the MyPlate meal doesn't necessarily show the importance of portion size, think of the plate as being small, as more of a salad plate than a dinner plate. "Go small" means creating smaller portion sizes and using smaller plates and utensils. If you let your kids choose their own portions, they might surprise you and choose much smaller portions than you would otherwise serve them. In making recommendations, the Dietary Guidelines use measurable terms, such as cups and ounces, to help people control their portion sizes and, thus, eat fewer extra calories. And while you probably don't intend to measure out your kids' food intake, the ability to "guesstimate" will help you and your family avoid overeating. "Go small" also applies when eating out. Most of the time restaurants serve very large portions. If eating at a fast-food restaurant, choose the smallest size you can (many will even allow adults to get kid-sized portions). If eating at a sit-down restaurant, consider asking the server to put half the meal in a to-go bag even before the food is served.

Nutrition Goals

Taking into account your family's typical eating patterns and those recommended for optimal health, set a few goals for what you would like to achieve over the next month. The first 2 goals I usually suggest are listed in the Family Fit Plan: Eat at least 3 dinners together per week and eat a total of at least 5 vegetables and fruits per day.

Physical Activity Recommendations

Based on the 2018 Physical Activity Guidelines Advisory Committee recommendations, adults should engage in 150 to 300 minutes per week of moderate to vigorous physical activity (or 75 minutes of vigorous-intensity physical activity), including at least 2 days per week of muscle-strengthening exercise. If that seems nearly impossible, don't worry. Benefits come from even lesser amounts of activity. For example, replacing sedentary behavior with light-intensity activity reduces the risk of heart disease, diabetes, and even death. There is no minimum amount of activity that must be achieved for benefits to occur. Some—even if just a little—is better than none.

For maximum benefits, kids aged 6 to 13 years should aim to do the following:

- Cardiovascular exercise, most if not all days, including at least 60 minutes of moderate to vigorous activity such as brisk walking, jogging, skipping rope, biking, or the movement portion of some sports.
- Muscle-strengthening exercise such as playing on playground equipment, climbing trees, playing tug-of-war, and more traditional strength training at least 3 days per week. If your child is interested in lifting weights, as long as he or she can follow directions on proper lifting to avoid injury, let him or her go for it! The American Academy of Pediatrics (AAP) recommends that a muscle-strengthening program targets all major muscle groups, starts with no load and incrementally progresses load once exercise technique is mastered, involves 2 to 3 sets of 8 to 15 repetitions, and lasts at least 8 weeks. If feasible, children who are highly motivated to participate in resistance training may benefit from a couple of sessions with a qualified exercise professional to learn good technique, reduce risk of injury, and get access to a safe and effective program.
- Bone-strengthening exercises such as jump rope and tumbling at least 3 days per week.

The good news is that some activities count toward 2 or all 3 of the cardiovascular, muscle strengthening, and bone strengthening requirements. For instance, running is both bone strengthening and cardiovascular, while an obstacle course is both cardiovascular and muscle strengthening. The 7-minute workout discussed later in the Family Fit Plan counts for all 3. Studies show that kids younger than 6 years need 3 hours or more of physical activity through-out the day, ideally in increments of at least 15 minutes of movement per hour while awake. Young kids love playing games like tag or climbing the monkey bars on the playground. Infants should be physically active several times per day, mostly through activities like tummy time and interactive floor-based play. For all children and adolescents, make sure that the activity is appropriate to a child's age, enjoyable, and varied.

Considerations as You Begin to Plan More Activity Into Your Days

As you help your family move more, consider your family's strengths that help make it easier to increase physical activity. For example, perhaps you all enjoy playing sports. Also think of weaknesses that make this more difficult. For example, perhaps you have a hectic work schedule and are too exhausted to exercise after a long day. Consider any opportunities (big or small!) that you might have to add more physical activity into your routine, as well as any threats that will make it more difficult. Refer back to your SWOT [strength, weakness, opportunities, and threat] analysis from Chapter 1. As you consider how you might add more activity into your days, keep the following considerations in mind:

- Kids who have parents who are active are more likely to be active themselves. Take the first step by finding a fun physical activity that you enjoy doing and make it a part of your daily life.
- Every family member may have a different level of interest and different skill level when it comes to physical activity. Help your kids find activities that they will enjoy, can do or learn to do, and will fit in to your family's schedule.
- More so than adults, the best types of physical activities for kids are those that are interesting and fun (although that is certainly important for adults too!). A child is much less likely than an adult to slog through another workout in hopes of achieving some health goal. Studies show that kids who participate in sports, have more outdoor time, and walk or ride their bike to and/or from school are most likely to meet physical activity guidelines. Consider adding physical activities that the whole family enjoys and can do together, or perhaps you can learn a new skill together.

I can guess what you're thinking—"Life is hectic! How are we going to do all of this?" The best chance for kids to meet physical activity guidelines is when the physical activity is built into the day. This is part of the reason school is such an ideal place for kids to get their daily 60 minutes of activity. If you have young children in preschool or child care, ask about opportunities and the schedule for active play and physical activities. If you have the option, consider choosing a preschool that prioritizes movement. Older kids might consider walking or biking to school, if that is a feasible option. If it is not, does the school offer a before-school activities program such as a running club or playground free play? How often does a child have physical education class? How long does it last, and how likely is it that a child will obtain moderate to vigorous amounts of activity in class? How many recess periods are in a day? For how long? What does the child typically do during recess? What opportunities are available in after-school programs? If your child has an interest in sports, how might the school help to fill in the gap? If you belong to a gym or health club, what options are available for your kids to be active while you work out? Or better yet, what opportunities are there for you all to be active together? Does a local facility offer family weight training or strengthening programs? What can family members do together or separately at home?

You might face some common challenges to starting and continuing physical activity, such as

✔ **Cost in both money and time.** As you may already well know, many youth activity programs require a significant parental financial and time investment.

✔ **Safety.** Access to safe play is limited for many children, especially those growing up in urban areas.

✔ **Time.** Many working families are not available to transport children to sports and other recreational activities. Many after-school and child care programs do not provide sufficient opportunities for children to attain adequate amounts of physical activity.

✔ **Physical health concerns.** Children with special needs, chronic conditions, and physical or behavioral limitations may face additional challenges in identifying activity programs that provide a child the best fit.

✔ **Competing priorities and interests.** If physical activity is not a priority for families and communities, it may not be a priority for children either. While many kids may start out active, as they get older, physical activity levels decrease. This is likely due to increased specialization for the most "elite" young athletes and a general dropping off of sports participation for everyone else. Adolescents are less likely to have physical education or physical activity opportunities as part of their everyday routines. A special focus on fun, engaging activity opportunities for teens are especially valuable.

✔ **Weather.** Unpleasant weather can disrupt the best plans for outdoor activity and keeps many kids inside and inactive. Have a backup plan that includes many indoor activities for bad-weather days (or months).

Take these potential challenges into account and brainstorm with your children how to overcome any barriers they may face in becoming more active.

A Note on Sports

Regardless of natural ability, level of competition, or physical or mental challenges, children benefit from participation in sports. Many participate for the pure joy and fun of the sport and friendly competition. Others play sports competitively in hopes of making the high school team, playing in college, or one day becoming a professional athlete. In any case, participation in sports offers children tremendous health, social, and developmental benefits. Children who play sports not only have a regular opportunity to engage in physical activity, but they also develop life skills including leadership, teamwork, self-discipline, cooperation, and how to experience both winning and losing with composure. Take care to help kids have an overall positive experience with sports. Repeated failures, criticism, excessive pressure, and negative peer interactions can leave a child permanently turned off to sports. Sometimes, parents need to step back from the game and refocus on what's important.

Now that you have a general sense of your and your family's baseline fitness (Chapter 2), and you know how much and what types of activity everyone *should* get and how much and what types everyone *actually does* get, it's a great time to set some activity-related SMART goals to achieve in the next month.

If you did any of the fitness assessments in Chapter 2, you could set a SMART goal to get better at 1 or more of them. For example, if you did the 1-mile walk/run in 18 minutes, you could set a SMART goal to complete 1 mile in 15 minutes when you repeat the test at the end of the month. The associated action plan might be to walk/run as fast as you reasonably can for 15 minutes at least 3 days per week, as well as to go for a speed walk around the block after dinner with a willing family member at least 2 days per week.

Play

Play is underestimated but incredibly important for kids (and adults too!). Today's kids have lost 12 hours per week of free time, with 25% less play and 50% fewer outdoor activities compared with children in the late 1970s. During free play, children learn problem-solving skills, practice leadership, burn energy, and develop important social and cognitive skills. The best play is child-directed, child-driven, and somewhat spontaneous. Overly scheduled children doing largely adult-directed activities have few opportunities for true play. Studies show that children who play together can create and explore their world while developing skills in sharing, decision-making, conflict resolution, teamwork, and language. Play also offers engaged parents a glimpse into a child's world. Bottom line: leave time for play (and resist the urge to overschedule).

Some of the ways the whole family can increase activity every day include

- Take a family walk after dinner. During each walk, try to cover the same ground in less time. When more challenge is needed, add distance to the walk.
- Walk the family dog together.
- Walk or bike the kids to school. Not only is it a great opportunity for physical activity and modeling a commitment to a healthy lifestyle, but it also gives you a few minutes of uninterrupted time together.
- Play a round of Simon Says or tag with your kids. They'll love it, and both you and your kids will be sure to get your hearts pumping.
- Instead of fast-forwarding the commercials when watching TV, mute the sound and have the whole family do curl-ups during the break. See how many you can do in total by the end of the show. Next week, try to do a few more. Continue to build up the number you can do.
- Play with your kids in child-driven and child-directed activities at least 10 minutes per day.

If you did not complete the family assessments, no problem. You can use the goals listed in the Family Fit Plan.

Ways to Make Physical Activity a Priority

Make an effort to add steps to your day in simple ways. For example, you can

- Take the stairs rather than the elevator or escalator whenever possible.
- Choose a farther-away spot in the parking lot when you go shopping.
- Stand rather than sit when you are at work.
- Schedule walking meetings with colleagues rather than sitting around a conference room.
- Walk over to talk with others at home or work rather than emailing, texting, or yelling for them.

Encourage your kids to do the same. For example, you can

- Suggest that teens have a friend over and go for a walk and talk together rather than texting each other for hours on end.
- Ask your kids to come talk to you face-to-face instead of screaming down the stairs when they are trying to get your attention.
- Tell your kids to walk or ride their bikes to visit a friend who lives down the street rather than giving them a ride.
- Have your toddler walk rather than pushing him or her in a stroller.

Help your kids learn to take advantage of opportunities when a few more steps can easily be added into the day.

Build Activity Into Your Schedule

Families who seem to always find the time to be active write their activities in each family member's calendar, making it part of a daily routine, and hold each other accountable to get those activities done. This does not mean that the activity has to last a long time, be very vigorous, or contribute to the overscheduling of a child's free time. It is best if it is fun. The sample family schedule in Figure 3.4 shows how activity is prioritized. If something comes up and a preplanned activity cannot be done, that is OK, but try to make sure that the activity happens another day and that not too many days in a row go by in which the routine is broken.

A Walking Plan

Most adults prefer walking over other forms of physical activity—and for good reason. Walking is an easy way to start and maintain a physically active lifestyle combining exercise, health promotion, fun, and transportation. It lets people be nurturing (eg, walking a dog or a baby in the stroller), social (when walking with friends), or meditative (when walking alone). It requires no special skills or equipment, carries a low risk of injury, and offers a lot of flexibility in choosing the right amount of effort and intensity. Start your walking plan by simply taking the first steps—even if just for a few minutes. Then, if you'd like, you can continue to improve your fitness by varying the frequency (how often), intensity (how hard), and time (how long).

Figure 3.4. A Schedule to Move

This is an example of a family that prioritizes physical activity in their family schedule.

	Monday	Tuesday	Wednesday	Thursday	Friday	Saturday	Sunday
Mom	Swim laps	7-minute workout, then 3-minute jump rope workout with son	"Walk to School Wednesday" with kids	7-minute workout, then 3-minute jump rope workout with son	Yoga	Run	Family activity
Dad	Lift weights in garage after work/ before dinner	Run after work/ before dinner	Lift weights in garage after work/ before dinner	Run after work/ before dinner	Off	Run	Family activity
Son	Basketball practice	3-minute jump rope workout with mom	"Walk to School Wednesday" Basketball practice	3-minute jump rope workout with mom Ride bike with friends	Ride bike with friends	Basketball game	Family activity
Daughter	Soccer practice	Before-school running club	"Walk to School Wednesday" Soccer practice	After-school jump rope	Before-school running club	Soccer game	Family activity
Family	10- to 15-minute family walk after dinner	10- to 15-minute family walk after dinner	10- to 15-minute family walk after dinner	10- to 15-minute family walk after dinner	10- to 15-minute family walk after dinner	Unscheduled	Alternating family fitness (hiking, basketball, rock climbing, biking, etc)

Get Fit With HIIT

High-intensity interval training (HIIT) has proven to be a highly effective and highly efficient way to boost physical fitness in a short period. HIIT sounds a little scary, but once you start you'll find that it isn't. HIIT is characterized by short periods of very high intensity exercise followed by periods of rest.

Give HIIT a try with the 7-minute workout (Figure 3.5). This workout requires little time or equipment but offers up big rewards in the form of improved cardiovascular fitness and muscle strength and endurance. Plus, kids 6 years and older can do it with you. Also check out the high-intensity aerobic interval walking and sprint interval walking plans in the Appendix.

Figure 3.5. The 7-Minute Workout
Each interval is 30 seconds, separated by 10 seconds of rest. You can time it yourself or use one of the many available 7-minute workout apps. Feel free to make modifications to make it fun and doable for your whole family.

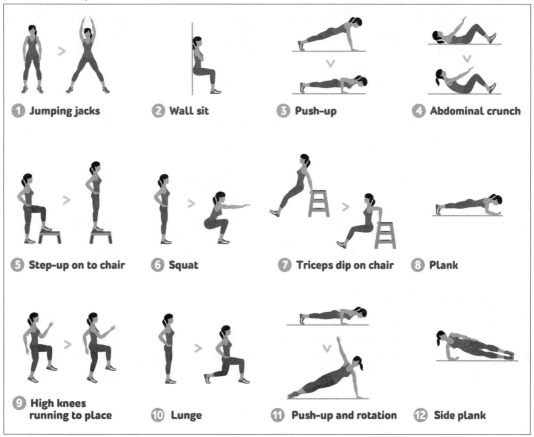

1. Jumping jacks
2. Wall sit
3. Push-up
4. Abdominal crunch
5. Step-up on to chair
6. Squat
7. Triceps dip on chair
8. Plank
9. High knees running to place
10. Lunge
11. Push-up and rotation
12. Side plank

Source [of workout]: American College of Sports Medicine

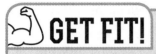

FAMILY 5K TRAINING PROGRAM FOR BEGINNERS

Make a plan to increase family fitness by signing up to complete an event together. Many 5Ks allow strollers, so even the youngest kids can join you. Don't worry about speed, per se, but more about the experience of accomplishment in setting a goal and achieving it together as a family.

Before each workout, warm up for 5 to 7 minutes; afterward, cool down for 2 to 3 minutes. It is OK to change the days to fit your schedule, but make sure you complete at least 3 walk/run sessions per week.

Week	Monday	Tuesday	Wednesday	Thursday	Friday	Saturday	Sunday
1	Walk 15 minutes	Walk/jog 1½ miles	Rest	Walk/jog 1½ miles	Rest	Walk/jog 30 minutes	Rest
2	Walk 15 minutes	Walk/jog 2 miles	XT	Walk/jog 1½ miles	Rest or yoga	Walk/jog 35 minutes	XT
3	Walk 15 minutes	Walk/jog 2½ miles	XT	Walk/jog 2 miles	Rest or yoga	Walk/jog 45 minutes	XT
4	Walk 15 minutes	Walk/jog 3 miles	XT	Walk/jog 2 miles	Rest or yoga	Rest	5K

Walk/jog = Alternate walking and running at a moderate pace. Initially jog for 1 to 2 minutes, followed by walking for 3 to 4 minutes. Each week, try to jog for 1 minute more and walk for 1 minute less. You could also substitute high-intensity aerobic interval walking (see Appendix).

XT = cross-training. On these days do any other physical activity that you'd like. These would be great days to build in the 7-minute workout or strength training.

Rest or yoga = These days can be rest days or consider incorporating family yoga into your routine (see Appendix).

Your Family 5K Training Plan

Did you set a SMART activity goal to participate in an event such as a 5K? Why not start a 4-week training program today and finish your 30-day Family Fit Plan with a celebratory 5K? Gather any willing family members and start the program shown in the GET FIT! "Family 5K Training Program for Beginners" Box today.

Choose Active Outings as a Way to Spend Time Together as a Family

Whether it is going for walks, learning a new skill together, or choosing activities such as rock climbing, hiking, or ice skating rather than going to a movie or out to dinner, physical activities can be a great way to spend family time together and show kids that physical activity is a clear priority. This will make it more likely that they will continue to be physically active as they get older.

If you are looking for ways to be more active and meet new people, consider some of the following opportunities that are available in many communities throughout the United States:

- Stroller Strides (http://fit4mom.com/programs/stroller-strides). Founded by mom Lisa Druxman in 2001, Stroller Strides is a national franchise (now part of the larger Fit4Mom corporation) that helps new moms get and stay fit walking, jogging, and working out with their infants and toddlers. Stroller Strides is active in more than 2,000 communities across the United States.
- Walking school bus (www.walkingschoolbus.org). In an effort to counter the trend of kids who live less than a mile from school getting dropped off by busy parents rather than walking or riding to school, the walking school bus offers communities a safe alternative. A walking school bus is a group of kids, typically who live in the same neighborhood, walking to school with 1 or more adults who often take turns covering the walk. An increasing number of communities have jumped on board with this initiative. If you are interested in starting your own walking school bus, free online training is available at http://apps.saferoutesinfo.org/training/walking_school_bus/modules.cfm.
- Special Olympics (www.specialolympics.org). With chapters in communities in every state and more than 170 countries, the Special Olympics offers year-round sports and athletic competition in more than 30 sports for children and adults with intellectual disabilities. The focus is always on what the athletes can do, helping the athletes "discover new strengths and abilities, skill and success."
- Walk with a Doc (http://walkwithadoc.org). David Sabgir, MD, was a frustrated cardiologist, repeatedly giving his patients the same advice ("move more") but seeing little change. He rallied a few patients on a Saturday morning to walk together. It evolved into a movement in his hometown of Columbus, OH, and then spread to communities across the country

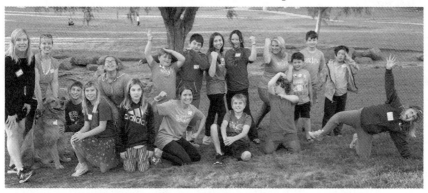

(300 and counting). Although many walks are more oriented toward adults, some, such as the one I lead in Carlsbad, CA, target kids and families.

Families in Carlsbad, CA, enjoy being active together each week at Walk with a Doc-Carlsbad. Walk with a Doc is a national program with hundreds of active chapters in communities across the United States.

Sleep

Sleep Recommendations

The American Academy of Sleep Medicine recommends the following amounts of sleep for optimal health:

- Infants younger than 4 months: No recommendation, as adequate sleep can be quite variable and does not seem to be associated with health outcomes
- Infants 4 to 12 months: 12 to 16 hours per 24 hours (including naps)
- Children 1 to 2 years: 11 to 14 hours per 24 hours (including naps)
- Children 3 to 5 years: 10 to 13 hours per 24 hours (including naps)
- Children 6 to 12 years: 9 to 12 hours per 24 hours

Of course, you can't *force* your child to sleep. What you can do is develop consistent bedtime routines and be consistent in enforcing them. Try the following 5Bs to help make this easier:

- ✔ **Bathe.** Taking a bath or shower before bed helps to calm the mind, which may make it easier to fall asleep.
- ✔ **Brush.** Brushing teeth right before bed not only improves oral hygiene and reduces cavities, but it also helps the brain to recognize a routine.
- ✔ **Book.** Reading nightly is a great routine to help build smarts and learn new things while it also calms the mind and makes it easier to fall asleep. (Note: Reading here means reading a book and does not include reading on a backlit screen or device. Studies show that the light from screens interferes with falling asleep.)
- ✔ **Breathe.** Take a few deep breaths. (More information on this and evolving these breaths to a calming exercise are covered in Chapter 5 [Week 2].)
- ✔ **Bed!** Time to go to sleep.

You can help your infant sleep better by following the approach outlined in Figure 3.6. To help yourself sleep better, see the suggestions following Figure 3.6.

Sleep Goals

How would you like your or a family member's sleep to improve over the next month? Review the sleep logs you filled out in Chapter 2, and set a SMART goal. Or follow the goal that is already in the plan if it works for your family. Remember: Only set goals for things that *you* can control (eg, although you cannot make a toddler sleep better, you can take steps that set the stage for your child to get better sleep).

Figure 3.6. How to Improve Your Infant's Sleep

Bedtime Routines	Sleep Location and Behaviors	Night Waking
Consistent routine 30–45 minutes before bedtime. Choose calm bedtime activity. Do not feed as the last step before bed.	Best bedtime is 7:00–8:00 pm. Avoid stimulating environment at bedtime. Put to bed drowsy but awake by 4 months of age. After 1 month of age, allow infant time to self-soothe when put down to bed.	Avoid "dream" feeds after 4 months. Allow infant time to self-soothe when waking at night. Keep night interactions with infant boring. Avoid overnight feeds after 4 months of age.

Source: Adapted from Paul IM, Savage JS, Anzman-Frasca S, Marini ME, Mindell JA, Birch LL. INSIGHT responsive parenting intervention and infant sleep. *Pediatrics.* 2016;138(1):e20160762.

You might set a SMART goal for yourself to sleep 30 more minutes each night by the end of 30 days. To accomplish this, you can

❶ Follow the 5Bs routine when putting the kids to bed each night.
❷ Read a book in bed for 20 minutes before you want to fall asleep instead of looking at your smartphone or watching TV.

Screen Time

When kids are not at school (and in some cases, even when they are!), many are spending their extra time looking at screens. According to reports from Common Sense Media, kids 8 years and younger average 2 hours 19 minutes of screen time per day, while the average teen typically uses about 9 hours of media (TV, social media, internet, or texting) per day, not including for school or homework. Studies show that teens who spend more time on screens and less time on non-screen activities (eg, physical activity) have lower self-esteem, life satisfaction, and happiness than their less screen-addicted, more active peers. Adults also struggle with screen time. According to a Deloitte consumer survey, the average US consumer checks his or her smartphone 52 times per day.

Screen Time Recommendations

The AAP suggests the following recommendations:

- **Children younger than 18 months:** Avoid screen time, other than video chatting (eg, with grandparents).
- **Children 18 to 24 months:** Limit screen time. Ensure that your children will only be exposed to high-quality programming, and watch with them to help them understand what they are seeing.

- **Children 2 to 5 years:** Limit screen time to 1 hour or less per day of high-quality programs. Watch with your children to help them understand what they are seeing and learning.
- **Children 6 years+:** Limit screen time and enforce consistent rules on the quantity and types of media. Ensure that screen time does not interfere with quality sleep or adequate physical activity.

In addition, the AAP advises all family members to turn screens off during mealtimes and 30 to 60 minutes before bedtime. Also, to help support better sleep and closer monitoring of what your kids are doing, keep TVs and other screen devices outside of the bedroom.

Screen Time Goals

Did you log how much screen time everyone in your family has? The AAP encourages all families to develop a Family Media Use Plan (https://www.healthychildren.org/mediauseplan) to help get everyone in the family on the same page regarding screen time. Even if you haven't done this, you can set goals or use the goal in the Family Fit Plan.

For example, a SMART goal might be to eliminate devices at mealtime by the end of the 30 days. The following are possible action steps:

❶ Each night before dinner, place everyone's smartphones in a basket and store the basket out of sight.
❷ Sit at the table to eat dinner each night, and make sure that the TV, computers, tablets, and phones stay turned off.

Stress Management

Stress Management Recommendations

In *Reaching Teens: Strength-Based Communication Strategies to Build Resilience and Support Healthy Adolescent Development*, published by the AAP, editor Kenneth Ginsburg, MD, MS Ed, FAAP, FSAHM, offers teens an approach to developing a stress-management plan. This approach is adapted in the following content that you can apply to younger children and adults:

- **Tackle the problem.** First things first—identify the problem or stressor. What is triggering emotional eating? What is causing nervousness or anxiety? What is keeping you from being your most fit, healthy self, physically and mentally? Next, decide what to do about the problem. Can it be tackled head on and fixed? If so, make a list of the actions that need to be done in small, less overwhelming steps. Can it be avoided? If the problem arises in certain situations, perhaps avoiding those situations will make the stress go away. Is the stressor outside of your control? If so, can you let it go?

- **Take care of your body.** It turns out that exercise and meditation are 2 of the most effective strategies in managing stress. Both help to increase the focus and attention needed to tackle a problem. Eating in a healthful, balanced way as a source of energy and nourishment not only helps to improve overall health and well-being, but it also prevents the "hangry" feeling from going too long without food or guilt for using food to cope with stressors. Getting recommended levels—both in quantity and quality—of sleep helps improve our patience and overall frame of mind, making tackling or letting go of stressors easier to do.

- **Deal with emotions.** Stress can trigger overwhelming emotions such as anger, frustration, and sadness. Learning strategies that help release those emotions in a positive way can be life changing. Some strategies that older kids and adults can use are visualizing, pursuing hobbies, reading, journaling, art, talking with someone, screaming into a pillow, crying, or singing along to a song that resonates with the situation. Younger kids may have a difficult time naming their emotions. Help them to do so out loud. Remind them it is OK to feel sad or angry. Young kids often are able to manage stress through activities that they enjoy, such as play, drawing, or storytelling. Additionally, they, like all of us, can benefit from increasing mindfulness, using tools such as S.T.O.P. (Mindful Moment: "S.T.O.P." Box)

Mindful Moment: S.T.O.P.

When feeling stress, anger, or frustration, children and adults can benefit from learning and practicing a well-known mindfulness exercise known as S.T.O.P.

Stop what you are doing.

Take a deep breath. This grounds you and creates space between a stressful trigger and the reaction. Repeat the breath 2 to 4 times.

Observe what is happening. Notice thoughts and feelings as well as physical changes in the body.

Proceed. Now continue with what you were doing.

Stress Management Goals

Did your family members fill out the COPE questionnaire (see Chapter 2)? What did you discover? How would you like the stress in your life to be different? Would you like less of it? Or perhaps you would like to learn more effective ways to help manage it? Maybe it's not your stress that worries you at all but that of a child or loved one. Set a SMART goal to help. Then list 2 or 3 action steps you can take to make progress toward your goal, such as in the example that follows:

SMART Goal

By the end of 30 days, I would like regular meditation to be a part of my stress management plan OR to help my child better manage stress, I am going to model positive coping strategies.

Action Steps

❶ Learn how to meditate.
❷ Practice meditation for 10 minutes each day before bed.

Pulling It All Together: Your Family Fit Plan

Use the form from Figure 3.7 (and Appendix) to outline your Family Fit Plan and develop SMART goals and actions for each of the 5 key areas (nutrition, physical activity, sleep, screen time, and stress management).

Figure 3.7. Your Family Fit Plan

THE _____ FAMILY FIT PLAN			
Our "Why":			
Our Vision:			

	SMART Goal 1	Action 1	Action 2	Action 3
Nutrition				
	SMART Goal 2	Action 1	Action 2	Action 3
	SMART Goal 3	Action 1	Action 2	Action 3
Physical activity	SMART Goal 1	Action 1	Action 2	Action 3
	SMART Goal 2	Action 1	Action 2	Action 3
	SMART Goal 3	Action 1	Action 2	Action 3

Figure 3.7. Your Family Fit Plan (*continued*)

	SMART Goal 1	Action 1	Action 2	Action 3
Sleep				
	SMART Goal 2	Action 1	Action 2	Action 3
	SMART Goal 3	Action 1	Action 2	Action 3
Screen time	SMART Goal 1	Action 1	Action 2	Action 3
	SMART Goal 2	Action 1	Action 2	Action 3
	SMART Goal 3	Action 1	Action 2	Action 3
Stress management	SMART Goal 1	Action 1	Action 2	Action 3
	SMART Goal 2	Action 1	Action 2	Action 3
	SMART Goal 3	Action 1	Action 2	Action 3

Figure 3.8 provides some tips that you might consider as you put together your Family Fit Plan.

Figure 3.8. Tips for Healthy Living by Age and Stage

Age	Top Tips
Infant (0–6 months)	• Ideally, breastfeed exclusively. Wait to introduce solid foods until a baby is 6 months old for exclusively breastfed infants, or between 4 and 6 months of age for formula-fed infants. • Breastfeeding moms: Eat a wide variety of foods of all flavors. Especially bitter vegetables (flavors transmit into breast milk). • Follow baby's cues. Key in to signs of hunger and fullness. • Start to establish regular daily routines, including for bedtime and reading books. • Playtime! Actively engage infants in playtime, including tummy time, for an hour a day or more. • Avoid screen time and limit television exposure.
Infant (6–12 months)	• Introduce a lot of different types of solids, waiting at least 3 to 5 days between introducing new flavors. Avoid cow's milk and honey until 1 year of age. Avoid sugary foods and juice. • Take advantage of immature taste buds with frequent exposure to bitter vegetables and other foods most toddlers tend to reject. This makes it more likely the infant will not reject the foods later. • Continue to follow baby's cues. Key in to signs of hunger and fullness. Avoid using food to comfort. • Keep track of infant's growth and weight gain. Expect birth weight to triple by the first birthday. • Encourage gross motor skills development. On average, a 6-month-old should sit alone, a 9-month-old pulls to stand and cruises, and a 1-year-old takes first steps. Most babies crawl between 6 and 9 months of age. • Follow a consistent bedtime routine and allow infant to self-soothe back to sleep from nighttime wakings. • Avoid screen time and limit television exposure.
Toddler (1–3 years)	• Recognize that neophobia (fear of trying new foods) is a normal developmental milestone. • Eat the same family meals together often. Give toddlers a perception of power through offering choice between 2 healthy options. • Keep mealtimes relaxing and enjoyable. Include at least 1 food a child will like and offer repeated exposures to foods a child does not like at first (it can take 15 or more tries before a child will accept a previously rejected food). • Avoid food rewards and bribes (eg, "eat your vegetables and then you can have dessert"). That makes the healthy food seem less appealing to the child and the unhealthy food more appealing. • Create plenty of opportunities for safe, active play. • Limit screen time exposure to video chats with relatives. • Follow a consistent bedtime routine. • Praise good behavior, limit the number of times you say "no," ignore unwanted behavior, and follow through on "threats."

Figure 3.8. Tips for Healthy Living by Age and Stage (*continued*)

Age	Top Tips
Preschool (3–5 years)	• Model healthy habits. • Increase accessibility and exposure to fruits and vegetables. You can "train the taste buds" to like new foods this way. • Involve children in food preparation. Kids love to eat what they help grow, choose, and cook. • Take advantage of the increasing influence of peers. Invite a child's friend who is an adventurous eater over for dinner. • Offer many opportunities for active play and building fundamental movement skills (eg, running, jumping, skipping, hopping, throwing, catching). • Limit screen time to less than 2 hours per day. Offer only educational or interactive programming. • Follow a consistent bedtime routine.
School age (5–12 years)	• Involve kids in growing, choosing, and preparing foods. They will be much more likely to eat them. • Teach simple nutrition principles. Kids this age are generally receptive to learning about why healthy choices are important. • Avoid sugary drinks. These drinks do not help kids feel full, add a lot of extra calories, and are harmful to health. • Capitalize on the "power of peers." Kids want to do what their friends are doing. • Participate in sports and other physical activities rooted in fun. Fun is a key predictor of whether kids will continue an activity. Avoid the urge to specialize in a single sport. • Develop and enforce a Family Media Use Plan, including limits to screen time and no screens during mealtimes or within 1 hour of bedtime. Do not allow screens in a child's bedroom. • Enforce a consistent bedtime and bedtime routine. • Talk about stressors and help kids learn positive coping strategies.

(continued)

Figure 3.8. Tips for Healthy Living by Age and Stage (continued)

Age	Top Tips
Adolescent (13–18 years)	• Learn to cook basic foods. This is an important life skill that will help improve nutrition intake. • Aim for eating 3 meals per day. Skipping meals is associated with decreased nutritional status. • Get enough sleep. • Eat family meals ideally at least 3 times per week. Not only does this offer improved nutrition, but it also leads to less risk-taking behavior. • Make time for fitness. Physical activity often drops off in adolescence, especially for girls. • Engage a teen in developing your Family Media Use Plan and gain buy-in for creating limits around screen time. Do not allow screens at mealtimes or within 1 hour of bed. Store phones and devices outside the teen's room at night. • Help teens identify and respond to stressors using positive coping strategies (eg, exercise, meditation, journaling).
Adults/ Parents	• Model healthy eating practices, including having a positive relationship with food and avoiding dieting. • Stock the home with many healthy food options and limit unhealthy options. Avoid the urge to hide unhealthy foods from the kids. Instead, plan desserts or eating out into the schedule. • Plan meals in advance and post the menu in a visible location. • Schedule family meals as often as possible and no fewer than 3 times per week. Turn off the electronic devices during mealtimes and use the time to connect with each other. • Model a physically active lifestyle, and support and encourage the kids to find physical activities that they enjoy. Help arrange for them to be able to get there to participate. • Follow your Family Media Use Plan yourself, holding yourself accountable for screen time limits. • Maintain a consistent bedtime and follow a bedtime routine to improve your sleep. • Identify and respond to stressors using positive coping strategies (eg, exercise, meditation, journaling).
Special notes for pregnant women	• Aim to gain the healthiest amount of weight (25 to 35 lb if body mass index [BMI] is less than 25 to start; 15 to 25 lb if BMI is 25 to 30; 11 to 20 lb if BMI is equal to or greater than 30). • Eat for 1⅕ people, not for 2. Calorie needs do not increase in the first trimester and go up by just 350 kcal in the second and 450 kcal in the third. • Eat a balanced and highly varied nutritious diet, including any needed supplements (eg, folic acid, iron, DHA). • Prepare for a successful breastfeeding experience. • Aim for at least 150 minutes of physical activity each week.

Creating Your Family's Schedule

By getting into the habit of incorporating new behaviors into your flow of daily living, you increase the chances that they will stick. You also can see how feasible your SMART goals and actions are once you try to incorporate them into your day. Most people's lives are full, so plugging in these new routines might mean having to take out some old ones, with particular attention to those habits that might get in the way of achieving your SMART goals (eg, extra screen time). But we don't want the changes to be too drastic or to make too many changes all at once, because that decreases the chances you'll be able to stick with the plan. Start small and make changes where they can fit for now. The Family Fit Plan is meant to be repeated, with progressively more changes that soon become part of your normal routine.

As you focus on family routines, at first you may find some resistance to change. But don't worry; if you stick with it, you will find that the changes become easier and the rest of the family begins to accept the new routines. Plus, children thrive on routines. Instead of coercing, bribing, or begging your children to make changes such as eating vegetables, getting exercise, going to bed on time, or better controlling their tantrums (good luck), you can instead adjust their routines in a way that sets the stage for them to do all of these things—without the battles.

Start with a quick consideration of your current daily routine. What parts of your routine do you love? Leave those pieces in place. What parts do you hate? Can you adjust them to make the day flow more smoothly? Can you make room for family dinners most of the time, 10 minutes of exercise each day, and a bedtime routine (for adults, too; check out the Did You Know? "Adults Need a Regular Bedtime Too" Box for more). These 3 pieces in your routine alone will boost your family's fitness significantly.

DID YOU KNOW

ADULTS NEED A REGULAR BEDTIME TOO
Consistent bedtime routines are not just for kids. New research shows that adults who consistently go to sleep and wake up at the same time have improved health outcomes, including decreased risk of cardiovascular disease, high blood pressure, obesity, and diabetes. In addition, adults who follow a consistent sleep-wake cycle are more physically active, more awake and alert during the day, and sleep longer at night than those who have inconsistent asleep and awake times. Although it already was well understood that very short and long sleep durations and poor sleep quality are associated with worsened health outcomes, studies show evidence to support the importance of a regular bedtime in promoting adult health.

Use the sample family schedule in Figure 3.9 to help you come up with ideas of what routine will work best for you and will fit your family's schedule. Write down your daily schedule, including time for eating, exercising, spending time with your family, and bedtime. For a toddler or preschooler, you can use the same figure and tweak it based on your child's schedule. Ideally, your kids will buy into the change, but if they don't, you can use your authority as parent to enforce the routine. Just do your best to get the full support of other adult family members who can help (rather than hinder) you in carrying it out.

Figure 3.9. Sample Family Schedule

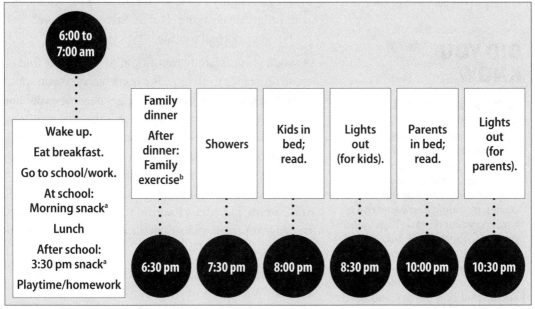

[a] Setting specific times for snacks helps to minimize grazing throughout the day and makes it easier to redirect a child who is always hungry to wait for scheduled snack times and mealtimes. Kids will actually be hungry at mealtimes and more likely to eat the food that is on the menu for that day. To minimize the amount of processed foods that kids eat, provide snacks made up mostly of fruits and/or vegetables whenever possible.

[b] Family exercise can be any type of physical activity the family does together. To make it more fun, you might consider having a "Sunday Fun Day" where family members take turns choosing a physical activity to do together. For example, 1 month's rotation in our family includes family P-I-G (basketball game), pickup soccer, hiking a local path, and going to a rock wall.

Family Meeting: SMART Goals and Action Steps

As you incorporate new routines into your family schedule, make sure to prioritize the weekly family meeting so you can check in with each other and plan for the upcoming week. Mark the meeting day and time on your family calendar and make sure that everyone is able to participate. The focus of the fourth family meeting is to put together your Family Fit Plan with SMART goals and action steps.

✔ Open the meeting by asking your kids what they already know about goals. Have they ever set a goal and achieved it? How did that feel? Do they have any personal goals that they are working on right now?

✔ Share that the purpose of the meeting is to set goals for the Family Fit Plan. You will decide what your family goals are, some actions you can take to accomplish these goals, and your new family schedule.

✔ **Activity for the week:** Discuss each of the 5 behaviors in turn, referring back to your starting line assessment from Chapter 2.

- **Nutrition:** Discuss food logs and create a goal with action steps.
- **Physical activity:** Discuss your activity log or fitness evaluation and create a goal with action steps.
- **Sleep:** Look at your family's sleep habits and create a goal with action steps.
- **Screen time:** Look at the Media Use Calculator or log and create a goal with action steps.
- **Stress:** Look at the stress questionnaire and create a goal with actions steps.

Write down your goals and action steps using the template in Figure 3.7. Alternately, you can simply use the outlined Family Fit Plan SMART goals and action steps (Figure 3.1) if they apply well to your family.

✔ **Activity for the week:** Create a schedule so that you can put this plan into action.

- Take a look at your current schedule and see what you need to add to or take away from it.
- Create a new family schedule using blank paper or a weekly calendar created for this purpose.

✔ **Closing family activity:** Ask each family member to share the goal he or she is most excited to work on, which change to your routine will be the hardest, and which one will be easiest.

Part 2
The Family Fit Plan

The Family Fit Plan is based on the latest scientific evidence, experience with hundreds of patients and their families, advice from the American Academy of Pediatrics, and trial and error with my own kids and family. Too often, books and plans designed to help you improve your health, nutrition, or fitness are go-it-alone approaches. They are tailored to a highly motivated adult who wants to make a fairly drastic change in a short amount of time. The person starts, and sometimes finishes, the plan; things change for a while; but then, eventually, old habits creep back in and the person gives up. A few months later, the cycle repeats itself. This is not the fault of the person following the program. More often, it is a problem with the program.

Two major flaws in many programs are

1. they push changes that are not sustainable, and
2. they rely on a single person making a significant change without paying adequate attention to the strongest predictor of whether or not a behavior change sticks—social support.

This plan is different.

The Family Fit Plan will improve health and fitness for the whole family. But more important than any specific change that you and your family members might make, you will have fun together on this adventure. I hope that this experience strengthens the relationships that you have with your partner, children, and any other family or friends who share your home or experience with you. I know it has for my family. We now have more meaningful conversations and more fun at mealtimes, cook and exercise together more often (in many cases with the kids leading the charge), and have fewer battles about sleep, screen time, behavior, and other daily frustrations. We all think that we are a bit stronger and healthier, too.

For best results, follow the plan as a 4-week series without skipping a week, and complete as many of the activities as you feasibly can.

Week 1: A Nutrition and Mealtime Makeover   **Week 3: Outsmarting the 6 Ss**
Week 2: Mastering Mindfulness   **Week 4: Savoring and Celebrating Success**

Don't worry if you don't get to everything. It is better to make 1 change that you can stick to than to make many changes that are short lived. Each week's activities and suggestions build on the ones before them, providing you with the structure and tools you need to develop and implement a plan to help your family achieve your fitness and health goals.

Week 1: A Nutrition and Mealtime Makeover

Food writer Michael Pollan is well known for his nutrition wisdom. From his legendary food rules to live by ("Eat food. Not too much. Mostly plants.") and his many best-selling books, he has become a household name for many nutrition connoisseurs. Earlier in his career as a writer for The New York Times Magazine, he pondered all the conflicting nutrition studies and slick food marketing campaigns and how modern people should make sense of nutrition information. He reasoned that modern people should do it the same way that their ancestors did. In a 2009 article in The New York Times Magazine, he said, "We relied on culture, which is another way of saying: on the accumulated wisdom of the tribe. (Which is itself another way of saying: on your mom and your friends.) All of us carry around rules of thumb about eating that have been passed down in our families or plucked from the cultural conversation."

Our culture—the family and traditions we were raised in as well as the "new" family and traditions we practice as parents and the head of the household—heavily influences not only our food choices but also the approach we take to parenting and raising a healthy family.

As you prepare to start the Family Fit Plan with a nutrition and mealtime makeover, consider your current beliefs about food and nutrition and why you feel that way. How much do you know about nutrition? Where did you get that information? How does it shape the choices you make in feeding yourself and your family? How open are you to tweaking your approach?

Take a Responsive Parenting Approach to Food and Mealtimes

Over the course of this week and throughout the Family Fit Plan, we will practice a responsive parenting approach to food and mealtimes with the following real-life and research-tested strategies.

But what is responsive parenting? Parents generally follow 1 of 3 styles in raising their kids: authoritative (responsive), authoritarian, or permissive. Authoritative (responsive) parents show high warmth and high control. That is, they set structures and guidelines for their children but leave room for flexibility and negotiation. Children experience certain freedoms within well-described rules. With this strategy, the parent controls the big picture, but the child is given the flexibility and freedom to make some choices. This is in contrast to low warmth, high control (authoritarian) parents. Authoritarian parents set rules and guidelines for their children and tolerate very little flexibility. They emphasize obedience and often withhold love and warmth. High warmth, low control (permissive) parents have few or no rules for their children and make very few demands of their kids. They tend to shower their children with love and warmth. Consider your own childhood. Which parenting approach did your parents primarily use? What approach do you tend to use with your own kids?

Taking an authoritative (responsive) parenting approach leads to the best outcomes, including improved family relationships, child independence and competence, and better overall nutrition and health outcomes.

❶ Recognize signs of hunger and fullness, both in kids and in ourselves.
People eat for many reasons—hunger, stress, boredom, socializing, and more. Mindless and emotional eating is very common and counterproductive to good health and nutrition. An important focus of week 2 of the Family Fit Plan is helping kids learn to recognize their body's signs of hunger and fullness.

❷ Offer age-appropriate foods and portion sizes.
Parents tend to greatly overestimate the amount of food that a child needs for good health (see Figure 3.3 in Chapter 3 for general portion size information by age and stage). The good news is that when kids listen to their body's feelings of hunger and fullness, they tend to eat the right amount.

❸ Use food for hunger only and not as a reward or punishment or to soothe a distressed but not hungry child.
A classic example of what not to do (that most parents have done at least once or twice!) is to tell a child some variation of "Eat your vegetables or you'll get no dessert." In the short term, it works to get the kids to eat the vegetables; however, in the long run the consequence of this strategy is that not only do kids like the dessert more than the vegetables, but when a reward is given to eat certain foods, the kids come to dislike even more the food they had to eat to get the reward.

❹ Repeatedly expose the child to foods to promote acceptance.
It can take 15 to 20 (or more) tries to train a child's taste buds to like a food. Just because your child rejected a food once, twice, or 10 times, don't call that food off-limits. Just casually introduce it again.

❺ Recognize the importance of modeling healthy eating behaviors.
Kids pay close attention to what their parents are doing and are much more likely to eat healthfully and have a positive relationship with food and eating if their parents do.

❻ Share feeding responsibility.
Specifically, practice the "division of responsibility" principle; the parent controls what foods are offered, when, and where, and the child chooses which of those foods to eat and

how much. Don't cater to picky eating preferences, but also don't force a child to eat what you've offered. For many parents, following this principle feels counterintuitive and takes a lot of practice (which you will get a lot of over the next 4 weeks).

❼ **Establish routines and limits.**

Practice implementing the schedule you developed in Chapter 3. Kids will eat a wider variety of healthful foods and fewer junk foods when meals and snacks occur at regular, structured times and are eaten at the table with no other distractions.

A 5-Step Nutrition and Mealtime Makeover

Now, let's put all of this advice into action by getting started with your nutrition and mealtime makeover.

Step 1. Clean out the refrigerator, pantry, and countertop.

If you're like most people, you'd like to help your family eat better with minimal mealtime battles and food fights. One way to achieve this goal and minimize the conflict is to set the stage so healthy food is more available and make the unhealthy foods less available. Do this by clearing out the stuff you'd like to avoid and loading up with the good stuff.

Refrigerator

Clear out the refrigerator completely. Wipe the shelves and throw away the expired, rotten, or never-to-be-eaten foods. Keep in mind that you are more likely to eat what is easiest to find and you're more likely to forget about the food that is buried in the back of the refrigerator, in a drawer, or that requires a lot of preparation.

Then, strategically restock the refrigerator. Start by putting the not-so-healthy foods in the back of your refrigerator. This makes them harder to find and eat. And you might even forget about them. Put the fruits and vegetables on the main shelves, ideally already washed and ready to be eaten. When they are highly visible, it is more likely that they will be eaten. Make sure leftovers and anything likely to spoil soon are in an easy-to-see location so you don't forget about them. Limit the space allotted for drinks to milk, water, unsweetened tea, and other healthful beverages. Ideally, throw out juice, soda, and other sugary drinks. But if that's not possible, try to decrease consumption by keeping only single-serving amounts in the refrigerator. Repeat this step often to prevent food spoilage and keep your refrigerator clutter free.

Pantry

Similar to your refrigerator, clean your pantry by emptying out everything. Throw out whatever junk foods you can without causing major family strife. That's not to say you should never eat these foods; just don't keep them in your house. This way you have to plan ahead for your desserts and less-healthful splurges. This helps to cut down on emotional eating as well as mindless snacking. Throw away outdated food and packaged food that contains sugar as the first or second ingredient. Do the same with the high-sodium products such as chips and highly processed snack foods. It is OK to keep items that you can't toss because you need to use them occasionally, but when you restock the pantry, store them in harder-to-reach places.

Restock the pantry with foods like nuts and seeds (preferably unsalted or reduced salt); grains, especially whole grains like brown rice, quinoa, oatmeal, couscous, bulgur, and buckwheat; oils like olive oil and canola oil; and dried spices and herbs to help liven up your cooking. Spices and dried herbs generally have a shelf life of 1 to 2 years. Check the flavor and color of spices to see if they are still up to par to meet your cooking needs (expired spices won't make you sick, but they also won't be very flavorful).

Countertop

Don't underestimate the power of a pretty, uncluttered countertop with strategically placed fruit and vegetable bowls in nudging your family to eat healthier. Start your countertop cleanup by clearing off the countertops and kitchen table and relocating the paper, mail, magazines, and other "stuff" to a file box. Or create an organization system to minimize the clutter. Likewise, if kitchen appliances such as a blender, toaster, coffee maker, or other gadgets have filled your countertops, try to clear some shelf space for those you don't use almost every day. If a cookie jar, candy bowl, or other highly visible and not-so-healthy snack is on your kitchen table or countertop, now is a good time to get rid of it.

Wipe the counters and get ready to redecorate. Start with a bowl of fresh fruit. Place it in a highly trafficked area, and your family's fruit consumption will increase immediately. Next, get the kids onboard to help you plant a small indoor herb garden. It may be just a few staples like basil and oregano, or you could be more elaborate. Kids love to eat what they grow. This small and easy-to-care-for garden will increase healthy food consumption and help to liven up home-cooked meals. Finally, place a vase or 2 of fresh flowers on the kitchen counter and the kitchen table. The flowers will brighten up the kitchen and make it a more enjoyable place for the family to prepare food, eat meals, and spend time together.

Step 2. Plan for meals and snacks.

Now is the time to plan the meals and snacks for the week. Using a meal planner like the one shown in Figure 4.1 may help keep you organized (this template is also available in the Appendix).

Figure 4.1. Weekly Meal Planner

	Sun	Mon	Tue	Wed	Thu	Fri	Sat
Breakfast							
Lunch							
Dinner							
Snacks							
Notes							

As you're mapping out what to eat for the week, keep the following tips in mind:

- Incorporate items you already have at home.
- Although you should consider your and your family's food preferences, there is no need to cater to them. You will be making 1 meal for the whole family, not many separate variations to accommodate picky eaters.
- Build your meals ideas using the MyPlate recommendations at ChooseMyPlate.gov. Make sure that half of your foods are vegetables and fruits, about a quarter are lean protein, and about a quarter are whole grain. Include dairy or a dairy-substitute 2 to 3 times per day.
- For dinners, include 1 or 2 easy, go-to, staple meals that you already eat frequently (although add some vegetables and/or fruits if they aren't already part of this meal). Then search through some recipes to choose a couple of new meals that you'd like to try (see the Appendix for some ideas). Or check out online recipe sources like ChopChop Family (https://www.chopchopfamily.org/learn-to-cook/recipe), Epicurious (https://www.epicurious.com), and the US Department of Agriculture Mixing Bowl (https://whatscooking.fns.usda.gov).
- As you're choosing recipes, keep your schedule in mind and how much time you can spend making the meals. Consider preparing large batches to freeze in meal-size portions, and reheat a portion another day (see the KITCHEN HACKS "Batch Cook—Freeze—Reheat" Box). Plan to reinvent leftovers by adding a few additional ingredients here and removing a few there to create a whole new meal. For example, leftover vegetables and meats can work great in a frittata, soup or stew, stir fry, or quesadilla.
- It may not be realistic to have home-cooked meals every day. That is OK. If you eat out frequently, when possible get familiar with menus and nutrition content of the choices before you go. Many fast-food and quick-serve restaurants have nutrition information available online. Try to choose healthier options and skip the sugary drinks. Most restaurants serve too-big portions. Choose a meal to share or pack half to take home before you even start eating. Be very cautious about kids' menus. While many restaurants are starting to do better, much of the time kids menus are loaded with salt and sugar and lacking in nutritional value.

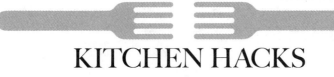

KITCHEN HACKS

Batch Cook—Freeze—Reheat

Save time during busy weeknights by preparing your meals for the week (or 2) in advance following this simple formula: batch cook—freeze—reheat.

Batch cook: Prepare 3 of the same (or similar) meal, 1 for this week, and 2 others to freeze and eat in future weeks. Cook your meats and pastas to nearly done but not all the way, as they will finish cooking when you reheat them. Make sure to cool the food before storing it in the refrigerator or freezer.

Freeze: Freeze any meals you do not plan to eat in the next day or 2. Types of meals that hold their taste and texture particularly well after freezing include soups and stews, casseroles, lasagna, and meat loaf, as they contain sauce or liquids that keep the food moist. Foods such as oatmeal, meatballs, stock, tomato sauce, and muffins also freeze well. Freeze liquids in a muffin tin, ice cube tray, or parchment-lined casserole dish first and, once frozen, transfer to an airtight freezer bag or freezer-safe plastic container. Label the bag or container with the date, name of the food or meal, and cooking or reheating instructions.

Reheat: Defrost frozen items in the refrigerator for about 24 hours prior to reheating to help retain taste and texture. (Exception: Skip the thawing for grains, as it will make them soggy. Also, you can go straight from freezer to oven for a casserole.) Then prepare the food according to the original baking instructions, to the desired temperature. Otherwise, reheat in the same method the food was originally cooked (eg, stove top, oven) for best results, although often a microwave will do. For more even reheating, arrange the food in a ring around the plate with a hole in the center.

Try out the batch cook—freeze—reheat method with our oatmeal recipe in the Appendix.

- Include breakfasts, lunches, snacks, and desserts in your planning. Figure 4.2 shows a sample 1-week menu using no-fuss staples and 30-minutes-or-less recipes that are included in this book. The sample 1-week meal plan uses the following MyPlate pattern:

  - **Breakfast:** protein/dairy, grain, fruit
  - **Lunch:** protein, grain, fruit, vegetable, dairy
  - **Dinner:** protein, grain, fruit, 2× vegetable, dairy
  - **Snack:** vegetable and/or fruit ± grain, protein, or dairy
  - **Reminder:** Everyone in the family can be offered the same foods, but let the kids choose how much they will eat. (See later in this chapter for more on portion size.)

- Once you have your plan for the week, make a list of items to pick up at the grocery store.

Figure 4.2. Sample 1-Week Meal Plan

	Sunday	Monday	Tuesday	Wednesday	Thursday	Friday	Saturday
Breakfast	Peanut butter and banana pancakes, fruit	Nutty oatmeal with fruit	Green chia smoothie	Cereal (<6 g sugar/ serving) and milk with fruit	Carbazu muffins	Yogurt and fruit parfait	Frittata muffins Whole wheat toast Halved grapes
Lunch	Tomato soup (Spinach) grilled cheese	Chicken sandwich Celery and cucumbers Apple	Peanut butter/ sunflower butter and banana sandwich Carrot sticks	Hard-boiled eggs Pita chips Black olives Halved grapes	Rainbow pinwheels Pineapple slices	Mean green pita pockets Blackberries	Tuna salad lettuce wraps Cheese and crackers Orange slices
Dinner	Barbeque chicken Corn on the cob Caesar salad Orange slices	Steamed fish with julienned vegetables Brown rice Roasted broccoli Fruit salad	"Taco Tuesday": make your own chicken or fish tacos Mango slices with spices Chips/pico de gallo/ guacamole	Spaghetti and spinach meatballs Salad Strawberries	Veggie-ful cheese- burgers on whole grain bun with tomato, romaine, and avocado Watermelon	Smiley face veggie pizza Salad mix Cantaloupe	Rosemary apricot pork sliders with apple cabbage slaw Tomato slices with (a little) salt
Snack	"Ants on a log" (celery, peanut butter, raisins)	Seaweed or kale chips	Homemade granola bar	Apples and peanut butter	Edamame and pita with hummus		Mozzarella cheese stick and black olives
Dessert	X	X	Frozen chocolate bananas	X	X	X	Peanut butter and honey crispy squares

Tips and Notes

- This plan shows variety to illustrate recipe ideas following MyPlate patterns. Recipes are included in the Appendix. You do not need to follow this exact plan. It is just intended to give you some ideas. It is OK to repeat meals, eat the same breakfast or lunch each day, swap a dinner for eating out, etc. The main thing is to keep in mind balancing your plate and trying to include ample vegetables and fruits in your day.
- Make it simple: batch cook chicken and oatmeal on the weekend and you will have breakfasts and lunches/dinners that you can vary throughout the week.
- Recommend: preplan 2 days per week that include desserts.
- Vegetarian protein options to substitute for meat/fish are included in the recipes.
- Customize your plan! For example, substitute alternate foods in the same food group to include family-favorite recipes and cultural staples in your meal plan.
- It is OK to substitute sunflower butter for peanut butter.

Step 3. Go grocery shopping.

Remember your list! Try your best to stick mostly to your grocery list when you are at the store. Time the trip so that you are not too hungry or too rushed. If you bring the kids along, prepare them ahead of time that you will not be buying any candy or junk food but that you would love if they would help you pick out 1 fruit and vegetable each (if they help you choose it, they are more likely to eat it later). When deciding what to buy, ignore front-of-package labels. Instead, get in the habit of reading the nutrition facts panel and ingredient lists to make sure you are getting high-quality food items. (The front-of-package label is usually trying to get you to think a food is much healthier than it is.) When choosing breads and other perishable items, check the expiration dates. Choose items at the back of the shelf (they are usually fresher than the ones placed at the front).

Step 4. Prepare and cook the foods.

Involve the kids at least somewhat in cooking the foods, as this will make it more likely they'll eat the food as well as learn important skills. Figure 4.3 provides ideas on how to engage your kids in cooking by age and stage. Yes, having the kids help may make it take longer, so you don't need to do this every time, but by doing it sometimes, you will move forward in your goal of having your kids eat more healthfully. You might consider batch cooking to save you time later. If you can prep vegetables and fruits now it will make it more likely that you and your family will eat them later, as it takes out the extra step of cleaning or cutting. Note, however, that once vegetables and fruits are cut, they do lose some of their nutritional value— but not that much. If the difference is between not eating them or eating them after they have been cut for a few days, you are much better off eating them when cut.

Figure 4.3. Kids in the Kitchen

Life Stage	Description	Kitchen Tasks
Infant	Once your child is sitting up well and has transitioned to the high chair, give your child a front row seat to watch you cook and also sample the foods you are making (make sure it's far enough away from the stove to be a splatter-free zone). Not only does this help make your child a more adventurous eater later on, but it also helps increase bonding. The modeling will make it more likely your child will want to help cook later on.	• Chief observer • Number 1 taster
Toddler	Toddlers love to explore with their hands. While they are often hesitant to try new foods, providing them with opportunities to help cook and to touch the food makes new foods seem a little less "strange" and ultimately increases the odds that they will try a taste.	• Sift. • Stir. • Paint pans/vegetables/chicken with oil using a pastry brush. • Play with real dough and cookie cutters as they would with Play-Doh (with supervision). • Pick fresh herbs from the garden/windowsill. • Help arrange foods into interesting shapes and designs.
Preschooler	Preschool-aged children are eager to help in the kitchen. Getting them involved in cooking is a great way to help them be less picky about their food, as they are likely to want to taste test while they help to cook. They will be much more likely to eat foods that they helped prepare.	• Rinse produce. • Measure dry ingredients. • Mix simple ingredients. • Cut soft fruits or vegetables with a dull knife or dough scraper. • Push down on the blender/food processor button. • Season foods with salt/pepper/herbs (with supervision). • Grease pan.
School-aged child	As fine motor skills, reading, and ability to follow instructions advance, school-aged kids can play an increasingly helpful role in the kitchen. The time spent together cooking also helps to create lasting memories, as cooking ignites the senses and those same smells, sounds, and tastes in the future will bring your child back to these moments together.	• Read recipe. • Peel vegetables. • Crack egg. • Prepare lettuce for salad. • Measure and mix dry and wet ingredients. • Open cans (with supervision).

(continued)

Figure 4.3. Kids in the Kitchen (*continued*)

Life Stage	Description	Kitchen Tasks
Adolescent	Teaching an adolescent how to cook—and better yet, helping an adolescent develop a true desire and joy in cooking—reaps huge benefits for the whole family. Not only can the adolescent help to make meals for the family and ease the weeknight scramble to put food on the table, but developing cooking skills will help your teen practice overall healthier eating habits and make him or her more self-sufficient when he or she goes off to college. When you cook together, you strengthen the bond with a child in a stage of life when parent-child relationships can often feel the most strained.	• Follow a simple recipe. • Boil pasta. • Chop vegetables. • Plan balanced meals.

Source: Adapted with permission from the American Academy of Pediatrics, *The Picky Eater Project: 6 Weeks to Happier, Healthier Family Mealtimes*. American Academy of Pediatrics; 2016.

Step 5. Eat together.

The most impactful step you can take as part of your Family Fit Plan is to make family dinners a priority. Studies show that kids who eat at least 3 meals per week with at least 1 adult family member have healthier overall eating habits. They eat more vegetables and fruits and fewer sugary drinks, sweets, and fried foods. They also do better in school, develop more advanced language skills, and are less likely to drink alcohol or experiment with other drugs as teenagers. Eating family meals together at least 3 times per week sets the stage for everything else that we cover in the coming weeks.

Finding Time to Eat Together

Many obstacles can get in the way of family mealtimes, such as work schedules, extracurricular school activities, homework, and sometimes being too tired to cook. Plan your schedules so that you make sure to eat meals together and say aloud that this is an important priority for your family. This sounds simple enough, but if you skip this step, the barriers to eating together will become overwhelming and you may fall into old habits.

Choose a time for dinner when most everyone can be there, even if that means waiting to eat dinner until 7:00 pm or eating earlier at 5:00 pm. Adjust snack times to make sure that everyone is hungry for dinner. If at all possible, make sure at least 1 parent is home for a sit-down dinner on most nights. Think twice before signing a child up for yet another activity that will extend into dinnertime. If eating dinner together won't work, perhaps there's another meal you can eat together so that your family can enjoy the benefits that come from regular family mealtimes.

What Do We Talk About?

What makes family mealtimes so important extends well beyond the nutritional quality of the food you eat. The shared time—free of devices and distractions—sets the stage for increasing connection through sharing experiences and stories with one another. The experiences often include conversations about the good and bad things that happened during the day for both parents and children. You can use this opportunity to help your children develop the skills they need to navigate through life's many challenges. It's okay to use the family mealtime to have unstructured conversations and go wherever the conversations may lead. You can also take a more guided approach to try to dig a little deeper in getting to know your kids and helping them get to know you better.

Psychologists Marshall P. Duke and Robyn Fivush found that children and adolescents who know a lot about their family—based on being able to answer many of the 20 questions on the "Do You Know…" scale (Figure 4.4)—are likely to have a higher sense of control, self-esteem, family functioning, and family cohesiveness and lower levels of anxiety and behavior problems. It is not the specific questions that offer up physical and mental health benefits but,

Figure 4.4. Do You Know? Scale: 20 Questions

1. Do you know how your parents met?
2. Do you know where your mother grew up?
3. Do you know where your father grew up?
4. Do you know where some of your grandparents grew up?
5. Do you know where some of your grandparents met?
6. Do you know where your parents were married?
7. Do you know what went on when you were being born?
8. Do you know the source of your name?
9. Do you know some things about what happened when your brothers or sisters were being born?
10. Do you know which person in your family you look most like?
11. Do you know which person in the family you act most like?
12. Do you know some of the illnesses and injuries that your parents experienced when they were younger?
13. Do you know some of the lessons that your parents learned from good or bad experiences?
14. Do you know some things that happened to your mom or dad when they were in school?
15. Do you know the national background of your family (eg, English, German, Russian)?
16. Do you know some of the jobs that your parents had when they were young?
17. Do you know some awards that your parents received when they were young?
18. Do you know the names of the schools that your mom went to?
19. Do you know the names of the schools that your dad went to?
20. Do you know about a relative whose face "froze" in a grumpy position because he or she did not smile enough?

Source: Printed with permission from Duke MP, Lazarus A, Fivush R. Knowledge of family history as a clinically useful index of psychological well-being and prognosis: A brief report. *Psychotherapy (Chic).* 2008;45(2):268-272.

rather, the family's sharing of stories. Researchers have found that the most impactful types of family stories are those referred to as the *oscillating family narrative*. This type of story shares the ups and downs the family has encountered but reveals that at the end, the family persevered. You might consider using one of your family mealtimes to see how many of the 20 questions your kids can answer. You might also quiz yourself; how many of the questions can you answer about your parents and grandparents?

You can also use family mealtimes to have a conversation about family traditions that you already have and why they are important. For example, are there certain foods you always eat at certain holidays, activities you do each summer, or a way that you celebrate birthdays or anniversaries? Are there stories you tell and retell time and again? These family traditions link generations together and reinforce a sense of belonging and a family bond. Perhaps with the start of your Family Fit Plan you may also have a new tradition you'd like to start.

A Time for Teaching Manners

I still remember the fancy etiquette class my grandma dragged my sister and me to when we were teenagers. The instructor's voice advising, "Bend at your knees and eaaaaaase into your seat," still sticks with my sister and me 25 years later. While we were just a tad defiant in that class (my guess is the etiquette teacher remembers us as fondly as we remember her), some of her teachings have stuck with me all this time. You probably don't need to ship your kids off to a class to learn manners. But you might find some value in teaching and enforcing some of the basic manners listed here. Family mealtimes are a great time to do this, with everyone "in it together," but keeping in mind that while we want to encourage a 9-month-old to eat with her hands, not so much for a teenager. While different cultures recognize different customs around mealtime manners, some general rules apply that you should feel free to adapt as needed to fit cultural norms. Also, even if you have a defiant teenager like I was, teenagers are still watching and learning from you as a model, even if it seems like they aren't.

- Always wash your hands before eating.
- Put your napkin in your lap first thing when you sit down at the table.
- Start eating when everyone else does or when the host (or parent) says it is OK to start.
- Keep both elbows off the table.
- Make an effort to talk to everyone at the table. But remember to chew with your mouth closed and wait to talk until after you've swallowed the food.
- When passing food around the table pass to the right (counterclockwise). If you'd like a dish at another time, ask politely for a person nearest a dish to please pass it, rather than reaching.

- Say positive things about the food, or nothing at all.
- Stay seated at the table until everyone is done eating or until you have been excused.
- Thank the host or whoever prepared the meal.
- Help clean up. Or at least offer.

How to Eat

Now that the food is ready and everyone is together at the table, it's time to notice how you eat. This might seem easy but there are some simple ways to keep track of the food your family eats. Help kids (and adults) practice listening to their bodies' cues for hunger and fullness. Avoid serving "family style," where family members can serve themselves from larger platters on the table. For most of us, if the food is there, we eat it, even if we aren't hungry. One way to counter this effect is to use smaller dishes and utensils so that less food is on the plate.

Let kids choose the portion size. Research supports that when given this opportunity, kids do a pretty good job of estimating the right amount (whereas adults are far more likely to give kids much more than they need). If the kids aren't old enough or you don't quite trust them to do this, make sure you offer them an age-appropriate amount. A general rule of thumb is that an appropriate serving size is about a tablespoon of food for every year in age, up to about 8 tablespoons (½ cup). Your kids will let you know if they are still hungry. Along these same lines, if a child refuses to eat, ask him or her, "Is your stomach full?" or "Are you still hungry?" This will help your child connect feelings of hunger and fullness with a decision to eat or not. Resist the urge to force your child to eat.

Slow down! Take one small bite at a time. Put the fork down between mouthfuls. Chew thoroughly before swallowing. Socialize during your meals and festivities. You can't eat and talk at the same time, so the more conversation there is, the slower you'll eat. At a family mealtime this week, have everyone count their chews before they swallow. Who chews the most? Who chews the least? See if you can all add 2 or 3 more chews to each bite.

Avoid commenting on which foods your kids choose to eat from the options you provide them. You have done your part by planning your meals ahead of time, ensuring that you are offering a variety of healthful foods, and getting everyone to sit down together at the table. Now let your family members do their parts by choosing what and how much they will eat without any parental interference. This will be incredibly difficult for many parents at first, but if you practice this consistently, you will find that over time, not only will family mealtimes become much more enjoyable, but your kids also will come to eat a wider variety of healthful foods.

Family Meeting: Nutrition and Mealtimes

Use this family meeting to launch your Family Fit Plan with your nutrition and mealtime makeover.

✔ Open the meeting by reviewing your nutrition goals and action steps.

✔ Share that the purpose of the meeting is to get ready for the coming week when you will make progress on your nutrition goals as you stock your kitchen with healthy foods, clear out the not-so-good stuff, and eat at least 3 home-cooked meals together.

✔ **Activity:** Make a list of the changes you will make this week and assign family members to the tasks. The recommended activities include

- Cleaning out the pantry and fridge, and decluttering the countertops.
- Planting a small indoor herb garden with the kids.
- Creating a weekly meal plan, making a grocery list based on your plan, and going to the store to be sure that you have all of the ingredients you need. Consider batch cooking.
- Involving the kids in the cooking of at least 1 meal this week.
- Eating family meals together at least 3 days this week.

✔ **Activity:** Make a list together of how you would like to celebrate your successes. Post this list on your refrigerator.

✔ **Activity for the week:** At each family meal, choose 1 or 2 of the questions on the "Do You Know?" scale to discuss. Share stories and examples that provide children with an oscillating family narrative (that is, share how family members faced a difficult situation and overcame challenges). Provide children with an opportunity to share experiences about themselves or experiences they have encountered in which they overcame a difficult challenge or had a positive outcome.

✔ **Activity for the week:** Go for a 5- to 10-minute walk after dinner most nights.

✔ **Closing family activity:** Close this week's meeting with a 5-minute family physical activity. If the weather allows, go for a walk together. Or turn on some music and have a 5-minute family dance party.

CHAPTER

5

Week 2: Mastering Mindfulness

To calm the inevitable chaos and frustration that comes with modern life and raising children, there is a clear role for mindfulness and meditation to improve the entire family's overall health, well-being, and fitness.

In adults, mindfulness meditation decreases depression, anxiety, and pain symptoms as much as medications. It also reduces psychological distress. The benefits for kids are likely the same, although, there is less available research to determine whether that's the case.

Mindfulness in the News

The harrowing story of a young soccer team and their coach trapped in a cave in Thailand rocked the world news in summer 2018. With seasonal flooding; a mysterious twisting, narrow abyss in the caves; and the knowledge that the boys had little water or food with them, everyone feared the worst. Except the worst didn't happen. Despite nearly 2 weeks of isolation, fear, darkness, and scarcity of resources, the team was rescued. All the children and their coach survived. The boys attributed their resilience to the skill of their coach, who was trained as a Buddhist monk, in helping them to stay calm and mindful. Each day of their seclusion, the team engaged in chanting and meditation.

During week 2 we will focus on mindfulness in 2 parts. The first part builds on what was covered in week 1 by continuing to increase mindfulness around mealtimes through increased awareness of the body's cues of hunger and fullness. We will discuss how to do this for kids of varying ages. The second part is increasing mindfulness through a more formal practice of meditation or yoga. You can find a practice that works well for your family and start to incorporate some form of meditation into your daily routine this week.

Mindfulness Around Mealtimes

Mindfulness refers to paying attention to the present moment, without being distracted by our thoughts, worries about the past, or lists of what we need to do next. Mindfulness around mealtimes and eating helps improve overall nutrition habits. For example, when we slow down and savor each bite—chewing slowly, experiencing the taste and texture of foods—we feel more satisfied and enjoy our food more, while eating less. What are the reasons people eat? Of course, hunger is one of the main reasons people eat. But it turns out that we eat for many other reasons as well. Following are a few common reasons people often mention when asked:

- Boredom.
- Sadness.
- Tastes good.
- Food is there.
- Celebrations and rewards.
- Social pressures and gatherings.
- Tradition, culture, ritual.

Are there other reasons you or your family members eat? Separate from merely providing sustenance, food is an important part of our lives. However, it is also important to be mindful about hunger and satiety cues to avoid overeating, especially in an environment that is dominated by ready access to highly palatable (ie, sweet and salty, which we are born liking), inexpensive, processed foods. We also are surrounded by many marketing and social triggers. When kids (and adults) develop mindfulness around eating, not only do they eat better, but they also begin to enjoy food more.

Our bodies tell us when we are hungry and when we have had enough. If we would only eat when we're hungry and stop when we're full, most of the time we would eat the right amount of food to maintain a healthy weight. But we don't do this—and so many of us can't do this—because for years we have not paid enough attention to our body's signals of hunger and fullness. Now as adults, we have many struggles with food, weight, and emotional eating. We can best serve our children by helping them avoid this predicament and teaching them how to better listen to their bodies.

Principles of Mindful Eating

Incorporate the following 11 practices into your daily routines to make eating fun without filling up on too many unhealthy foods. In addition, these practices will help empower your kids to make better choices, even when they are not with you.

❶ Teach your kids how to use the hunger scale (Figure 5.1). Have your children ask themselves before eating, "Am I hungry?" and before taking seconds, "Am I full?" When using the hunger scale, avoid the red zones (extremely hungry or overly stuffed). Instead, start eating around 3 or 4 (stomach growling) and stop eating around 5 or 6 (feel content but not uncomfortable).

Mindful eating is something that children can be taught, even when as young as 3 years old. For example, in one experiment, researchers taught preschoolers to pay attention to their own feelings of hunger and fullness by using a doll with a clear glass stomach. The adult showed the

Figure 5.1. The Hunger Scale

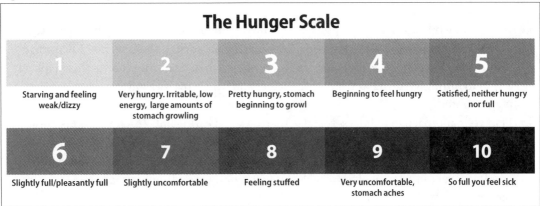

children the doll's stomach and then asked them to point to their own stomachs and say if they felt hungry or full. Next, they talked about what it feels like to be hungry and to be full. Then, the children fed the doll a small number of dried beans to show how eating fills up the stomach and how feelings of hunger would start to change. Afterward, the children were fed a snack and told to eat only until they felt full and then to stop eating. These children were able to eat based on hunger and stop eating when they were full, even when there was still more of the snack available.

❷ Use smaller dishes and utensils so that less food is on the plate and each bite is a smaller portion.

❸ Encourage portion control. Make it the norm to portion out snacks (versus sitting in front of the TV with the whole bag). Keep vegetables and fruits, such as baby carrots, apple slices, and edamame on hand for snacking. Another great tool for controlling the portion size of a snack is using snack-sized baggies.

❹ Let kids choose the portion size. As discussed during week 1, research supports that when given this opportunity, kids do a pretty good job of estimating the right amount to take (whereas adults are far more likely to give them much more than they need).

❺ Slow down. If your child finishes everything and asks for more food, ask your child where he or she falls on the hunger scale. Remind your child that it can take 20 minutes to feel full after eating and maybe it hasn't been enough time for your child's stomach to signal to the brain that he or she has had enough. Allow your child to take more food if he or she is still hungry.

❻ Identify and remove triggers. Remove temptations in your physical environment, such as filled candy dishes in the living room and cookie jars in the kitchen, that encourage family members to eat when they aren't hungry. Get rid of juice boxes, sodas, and other sugary drinks. Notice your and your family members' triggers and devise a plan to cope with them in a healthy way.

7 Be present while eating. In other words, when you are eating don't do anything else, such as reading, homework, watching television, texting, or surfing the Internet. Encourage family members to do most of their eating in the kitchen or dining room. This helps put a stop to mindless eating in front of the television, while playing video games, or when trying to study.

8 Plan your approach to holidays, social gatherings, and eating out. Teach your kids polite ways to decline food, have a plan for desserts, graciously decline offers to bring home leftovers, and, whenever possible, discuss and decide ahead of time what to eat when eating out. If you eat out often, look into healthier menu options and choose those most of the time.

9 Encourage physical activity. Not only will children burn off energy and have fun, but they will not be inside snacking.

10 Set a good example. When you're bored, angry, tired, or stressed, rather than food, turn to such alternatives as a quick walk, music, a bath, or a phone call with a friend. Or, grab the kids and get in a quick workout together. It could just be running up and down the stairs for a minute, or our handy 3-minute jump rope workout (see GET FIT! "3-Minute Jump Rope Workout" Box). This type of quick activity not only offers significant health benefits, but it also helps to calm and focus the mind.

11 Self-monitor nutrition and physical activity. The best way to increase awareness around nutrition and physical activity is to track yourself. Use the Family Fit Tracker (Figure 5.2 and in the Appendix), your smartphone camera, or your own favorite tools and apps to self-monitor your own food and activity patterns this week and, to the extent possible, that of your kids. Older kids and teens can do this for themselves.

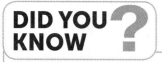

DID YOU KNOW ?

Studies suggest that 1 minute of all-out cardiovascular exercise offers similar benefits as 45 minutes of moderate exercise.

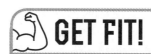

GET FIT! 3-MINUTE JUMP ROPE WORKOUT

Jumping rope isn't just for kids and elite athletes! It's one of the best physical activities anyone can do to improve cardiovascular endurance and bone strength. Grab the kids and try out our 3-minute jump rope workout (see Appendix) to de-stress, sharpen mental focus, and get fit with minimal investment of time and money.

Figure 5.2. The Family Fit Tracker

HEALTH TRACKER

MONTH/YEAR: _____

		FOOD	PHYSICAL ACTIVITY
MONDAY	B		
	L		
	D		
	S		
TUESDAY	B		
	L		
	D		
	S		
WEDNESDAY	B		
	L		
	D		
	S		
THURSDAY	B		
	L		
	D		
	S		
FRIDAY	B		
	L		
	D		
	S		
SATURDAY	B		
	L		
	D		
	S		
SUNDAY	B		
	L		
	D		
	S		

The 11 principles of mindful eating apply to the whole family. In particular, practicing the division of responsibility—you decide what foods are offered, when, and where, but your child decides what and how much of it to eat—is critical at all ages. However, the recommendations by age and stage described as follows may also be useful in helping your children use internal cues of hunger and fullness when deciding how much to eat:

Infant (0 to 1 Year)

Use your baby's signals of hunger (and not a specific amount of time for the feeding or a specified amount of formula) to decide when and how much to feed him or her. Some common signs of hunger include whimpering or smacking the lips, waking and looking alert, putting hands toward the mouth, making sucking motions, and becoming more active. If your baby becomes fussy with feeding, slows down sucking, falls asleep, or spits out or refuses the nipples, chances are your baby is full.

Toddler (1 to 3 Years)

Offer children a couple of healthy food choices (eg, broccoli or carrots). Let them feed themselves as much as they would like. Sure, it's messier than if you do it, but it helps them develop fine motor skills and a better sense of control over what and how much they eat. If your toddler doesn't want to try a new food, let it be okay. Reminders such as "Don't forget to eat your apples" are more effective at encouraging intake (if your child is still hungry) than coercive ones such as "I told you to eat the apple."

Preschooler (3 to 5 Years)

The preschool years are when many children lose the ability to use hunger and fullness cues to control food intake. This was demonstrated in a simple experiment. Children 3½ and 5 years old were given a heaping serving of macaroni and cheese versus a standard portion. The younger kids ate the standard amount regardless of how much food was presented to them. But for the 5-year-olds, the bigger the portion, the more they ate. The good news is that you can "retrain their brains." Talk to your child about what it feels like to be hungry and what it feels like to be full. Even preschoolers can start to learn to use the hunger scale.

School Age (5 to 11 Years)

As your child ventures off into elementary school, peers and the school environment become increasingly influential. By now, eating habits are well established and most kids don't do that great of a job regulating food intake based on hunger and satiety, especially if there is a lot of junk food available. But children at this age can learn to better listen to their bodies. For example, school-aged children who are overweight tend to eat faster and take bigger bites. After an intervention that included education, modeling, and practice, kids learned to chew more thoroughly and set food down between bites.

Adolescent (12+ Years)

The adolescent diet typically includes a lot of snacks and meals of processed, sugary, and salty foods and drinks enjoyed with friends. Teens can eat smarter by making a concerted effort to be mindful about food and beverage choices. In addition to eating better-quality foods, they can try to eat at specified times during the day, portion out snacks rather than eating directly from the box or the bag, avoid eating while distracted (eg, video games, social media, TV, studying) and be cautious about drinking too many calories (calories from drinks are less likely to contribute to feeling full).

Mindfulness Training

When the mindfulness approach extends beyond nutrition and mealtimes, it can help kids improve behavior, memories, and test scores while reducing anxiety, aggression, and stress, and improve overall happiness. Children can learn mindfulness at a young age. In fact, a fun way to encourage activity and increase mindfulness is to incorporate a little bit of yoga into your family's routines. Even toddlers can pick up some of the poses (see Mindful Moment: "Animal-Inspired Yoga" Box).

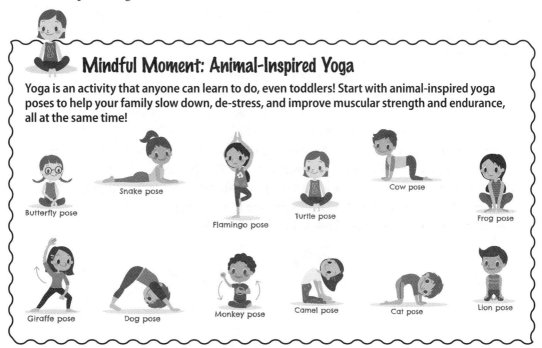

Mindful Moment: Animal-Inspired Yoga

Yoga is an activity that anyone can learn to do, even toddlers! Start with animal-inspired yoga poses to help your family slow down, de-stress, and improve muscular strength and endurance, all at the same time!

Butterfly pose

Snake pose

Flamingo pose

Turtle pose

Cow pose

Frog pose

Giraffe pose

Dog pose

Monkey pose

Camel pose

Cat pose

Lion pose

When parents and kids together make a point to practice mindfulness regularly, the behavior becomes a habit that can stay with kids even as they grow up and go off on their own as college students and later as independent adults. While this book serves only as an introduction to incorporating mindfulness into daily life, many resources are available for families who wish to learn and practice more. The Family Fit Plan mindfulness training focuses on developing 3 key skills that, when practiced regularly, will help the whole family improve nutrition, activity, sleep, and stress management. These skills are *awareness, tactical pause,* and *strength spotting.*

Awareness

We've talked about awareness when it comes to the importance of self-monitoring nutrition intake and physical activity. Awareness, whether it is of our habits, strengths, weaknesses, or emotions, is an important first step to making any behavior change. But awareness, along with *noticing,* is also important to help us enjoy life more, strengthen our relationships with people whom we care about the most, and avoid mistakes. Although many parents (myself included) pride ourselves on an ability to multitask, mindfulness training reminds us to slow down and pay attention, especially when we are doing very important tasks and when we are spending quality time with our families. As mindfulness guru Amit Ray said, "Life is a dance. Mindfulness is witnessing that dance." This week, help your family become better witnesses to the dance by trying out 1 or more of the following awareness-building activities:

✔ **The rainforest romp.** Invite the kids to join you on a rainforest romp. Go for a walk and ask the kids to notice as many birds, animals, bugs, and insects as they can. Look for anything that walks, runs, crawls, swims, or moves in some other way. See if you can find any creatures that you've never noticed in the past.

✔ **Taste test.** Invite the kids to join you in a taste-testing game. Try this out with the dips taste test experiment in the LET'S EXPERIMENT "Taste Test! Dips" Box. You also can try blindfold taste tests in which you blindfold each child and instruct him or her to use the senses of touch, smell, sound, and taste to try to identify a food.

✔ **Heartbeat exercise.** Together with the kids, jump up and down or do jumping jacks for 1 minute. Then sit down, close your eyes, and put your hand over your heart. Pay attention only to your heartbeat. What does it feel like?

LET'S EXPERIMENT: Taste Test! Dips

Nothing is quite as effective at helping kids be adventurous and try new foods than an experiment. The very nature of an experiment is that we don't know what is going to happen, butwe are willing to make an educated guess and give it a try. This offers a low-key way for a child to choose to try a new food. Who knows whether the child will like it or not? And whatever the outcome is…that's OK because we are just testing an idea out to see what happens. This experiment includes tasting a few different types of raw vegetables in 3 different types of dip to see what taste a child likes best—and if what kids like after trying is the same or different as what they thought they'd like before trying. Kids also get to practice using all of their senses when trying a vegetable. This mindful eating skill will help them learn to savor foods.

Try the following taste test experiment:

Step 1: Purchase, clean, and cut a variety of raw vegetables. The vegetables might include carrots, cucumbers, broccoli, zucchini, olives, or some other vegetable you or your children would like to try. Include 2 to 5 vegetables in your experiment. Write the name of each vegetable you chose under the "vegetable" column below.

Step 2: Before tasting any of the vegetables, ask your children to rate how much they think they will like each raw vegetable on a scale of 2 thumbs up 👍👍 (love it!), 1 thumb down 👎 and 1 thumb up 👍 (it's OK), or 2 thumbs down 👎👎 (don't like it).

Step 3: Then ask your children to rate which way they think they will like each vegetable best— raw or with dip 1, 2, or 3. Draw a star in that column.

Step 4: Together with your children, make each of the dip variations in the recipe "Creamy White Bean Hummus" in the Appendix.

Step 5: Start with the first vegetable on your list. Ask your child to use all his senses to describe how the raw vegetable looks, feels, smells, sounds, and tastes. Then ask him to give it a rating (two thumbs up, one thumb up and one down, two thumbs down). Note this in the "Raw Rating" column. How does this compare to how he thought he would like the vegetable before tasting it? Repeat this step with the other vegetables.

Step 6: Now try each vegetable with dip 1, dip 2, and dip 3. Ask your child which way he likes each vegetable best. Note this with a heart. Is it the same one he thought he would like best (the one he starred in Step 3)?

Step 7: Compare how much your children actually liked each vegetable and dip with how they thought they would like each one. What was surprising?

Vegetable	Before Rating	Raw Rating	Dip 1 (Creamy White Bean Hummus)	Dip 2 (Rosemary and Sun-dried Tomato)	Dip 3 (Green Onion and Olive)
eg, carrots	👎👍	👍👍	★		♥

Tactical Pause

Tactical pause is a term borrowed from the military that describes the space between an action and a reaction. A tactical pause is taking the time to consider a critical decision before acting on it. It is the pause before yelling at someone who did something aggravating. It is waiting to consider hunger before eating the delicious food placed in a bowl in front of you. In stressful or emotional situations, incorporating a tactical pause can help all of us better manage stress and think carefully about our choices and actions. In mindfulness training, kids learn to create this space and use a tactical pause to their advantage through mindful breathing (see Mindful Moment: "Mindful Breathing" Box).

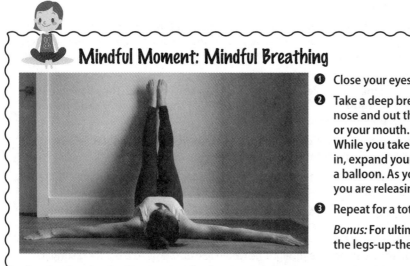

Mindful Moment: Mindful Breathing

❶ Close your eyes.

❷ Take a deep breath in through your nose and out through your nose or your mouth. Notice each breath. While you take the deep breaths in, expand your stomach as if it is a balloon. As you exhale, imagine you are releasing air from a balloon.

❸ Repeat for a total of 10 breaths.

Bonus: For ultimate calming, do this in the legs-up-the-wall yoga position.

Start by incorporating mindful breathing into the bedtime routine, adding a fifth "B" to the 4 Bs bedtime routine of bath, brush, book, and bed. Make it bath, brush, book, breathe, and bed. By teaching your kids this breathing skill in a low-stress situation (trying to fall asleep), it will be easier for them to use it naturally in higher-stress situations (those that require the tactical pause). Adults who would like to further incorporate mindfulness meditation may enjoy the free resources available from UCLA at http://marc.ucla.edu/mindful-meditations.

The STOP mindfulness activity described in Chapter 3 is another tool for practicing the tactical pause: Stop what you are doing. Take a deep breath. Observe what is happening. Proceed.

Strength Spotting

Martin Seligman, the founder of positive psychology, observed that "raising children, I realized, is vastly more than fixing what is wrong with them. It is about identifying and nurturing their strongest qualities, what they own and are best at, and helping them find niches in which they can best live out these strengths." It is human nature to pay more attention to negative experiences and emotions. However, just like we can train our taste buds to like new foods, we can also train our brains to direct more attention to positive experiences and emotions, especially when it comes to helping our children thrive. Teach kids to spot their own and other people's strengths. One way to do this is by putting names to strengths. Peterson and Seligman described 24 strengths within 6 categories that form good character and citizenship. They termed this the *VIA Classification of Strengths* (more information is available at https://www.viacharacter.org).

- **Wisdom:** Creativity, curiosity, judgment, love-of-learning, perspective
- **Courage:** Bravery, honesty, perseverance, zest
- **Humanity:** Kindness, love, social intelligence
- **Justice:** Fairness, leadership, teamwork
- **Temperance:** Forgiveness, humility, prudence, self-regulation
- **Transcendence:** Appreciation of beauty, gratitude, hope, humor, spirituality

Discuss with your kids the meaning of each of these strengths. Then ask them what they think is their own greatest strength. What do they think are the top strengths for each family member? How might recognition of these strengths help your family reach your goals? If you're interested in learning more about your and your family's strengths, adults and children aged 10 to 17 years can take the adult or youth VIA survey free of charge at https://www.viacharacter.org.

Family Meeting: Mastering Mindfulness

During week 2, help everyone in your family incorporate more mindfulness into their daily routines.

✔ Open the meeting by reviewing your stress goals and action steps.

✔ Share that this week's focus is on mindfulness. Ask family members to share what the word *mindfulness* means to them. In what areas of their life do they think they would do better if they were more mindful?

✔ **Activity:** Choose 1 of the following activities to do during your family meeting:
- Introduce and discuss the hunger scale (Figure 5.1). (After the Family Meeting, refer to it throughout the week.)
- Complete the VIA character strengths survey (https://www.viacharacter.org).

✔ **Activity for the week:** Make plans to incorporate as many of the following Activities for the Week that you reasonably can:
- Self-monitor nutrition and physical activity using the Family Fit Tracker in Figure 5.2.
- Map out your weekly meal plan (see the Weekly Meal Planner and recipe ideas in the Appendix).
- Map out your weekly fitness plan (see the Family Fit Tracker in the Appendix).
- Map out and post your family schedule.
- Incorporate mindful breathing into your bedtime routine (see Mindful Moment: "Mindful Breathing" Box).
- Incorporate an awareness building activity (rainforest romp, blindfold taste test, or heartbeat exercise) into 1 day this week.
- Go for a 5- to 10-minute walk after dinner most nights.
- Try out the Taste Test! Dips Experiment.

✔ **Closing family activity:** Close this week's meeting by practicing together 1 of the following activities:
- The 3-minute jump rope workout (See GET FIT! "3-Minute Jump Rope Workout" Box.)
- Animal-inspired yoga (See Mindful Moment: "Animal-Inspired Yoga" Box.)
- Mindful breathing (See Mindful Moment: "Mindful Breathing" Box.)
- Legs-up-the-wall yoga position (See Mindful Moment: "Mindful Breathing" Box.)

Week 3: Outsmarting the 6 Ss

"All great changes are preceded by chaos," noted Deepak Chopra, author, physician, and mind-body guru. Now that you are halfway through your Family Fit Plan, perhaps you've encountered a little chaos as you've guided your family toward great change. Whatever you have experienced so far is OK and normal. Although the plan is organized as a 30-day/4-week program, it is OK to extend it to a longer period by spending more than 1 week completing each section, or you can take a pause. It is also OK to slow down and focus on just 1 area of change at a time.

If you feel that you have hit a wall or your family is not progressing the way that you had envisioned, you may be up against 1 or more of the 6 Ss: snacks, sweets, sugary drinks, screen time, sleep disruptors, and slick sales and marketing. This week we explore these hindrances along with strategies to recognize them and change course to avoid, or at least minimize, their effects.

Snacks

Snacks are everywhere, from playgroups and sports outings to the classroom and after-school programs. On a typical day, most kids are offered many snacks. It's a rare child who will turn one down. Too often, kids will get home from school, grab a bag of chips, and sit in front of the TV, on the computer, or with their smartphone and mindlessly eat until the bag is empty. Or sometimes they will graze all day long and then show up at mealtimes not hungry or uninterested in eating the balanced meal in front of them. The key to smart snacking is having a plan for *when/where/how* snacking occurs and *what* the snack is. Follow these 3 steps to help your children snack smarter:

❶ *Make snacks part of a routine.*

As you know already, kids thrive on routines. If you haven't done this already, incorporate a snacking routine into your day that follows a schedule. Set times for snacks, such as 10:30 am and 3:30 pm. This helps kids know when to expect to eat, which can help stop all-day grazing. If a child wants to eat before it is snack time, redirect and remind him or her when the next meal or snack will occur. When it is time for a snack, allow kids to use their own hunger cues to choose how much to eat. Of course, you have less control over snacks when the kids are outside the house, whether at school or with friends. Most schools and after-school programs follow a snack schedule. Help your kids pack healthy snacks, or if they are getting a snack at school, advocate that only healthy options be offered.

❷ Consider the serving size.

Have you ever looked at a nutrition label on a package of what you would consider junk food, only to be surprised that the food was not as unhealthy as you thought? Did you look at the serving size on the nutrition label and notice how many servings per container are in the package? It used to be that even packages that appeared to be 1 serving had a nutrition label showing the nutritional content for only a fraction of the container. For example, a 20-ounce bottle of soda had 2½ servings. A 3-ounce bag of chips contained 3 servings. Nutrition labels have been updated, and portion sizes on packages now are required to reflect a serving size that is more typical of what a person would eat or drink. For example, the nutrition label for that 20-ounce bottle of soda now shows the full number of calories and sugar in a whole bottle. This doesn't mean that a person *should* consume a whole bottle. The amount of food designated as 1 serving is based on the amount that people usually consume, which generally is a lot more than recommended. Figure 6.1 is a primer on changes to the nutrition label and how to read the updated label.

Figure 6.1. The New Nutrition Label

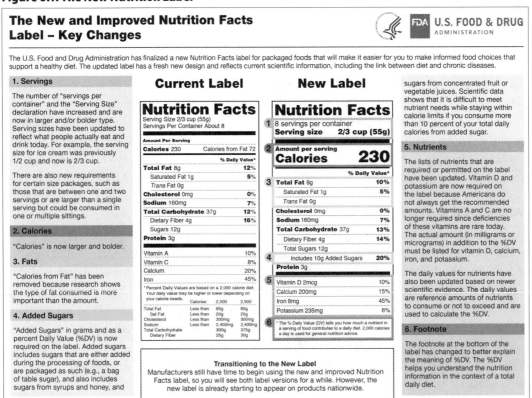

Source: Reprinted from https://www.fda.gov/downloads/food/labelingnutrition/ucm511646.pdf. Accessed March 10, 2019.

You can make portion control easier by purchasing snack foods that are inherently portion controlled, such as an apple or orange, cheese stick, prepackaged 1-ounce bag of mixed nuts, or a small box of raisins. Many packaged convenience foods, such as crackers and chips, also come in single-serving packages. You can also portion multi-serving snack foods into single-serving snack bags yourself or eat them only after putting them into a small snacking bowl. The LET'S EXPERIMENT "Portion Sizing Your Snacks" Box offers a family activity you can do to practice with portions.

LET'S EXPERIMENT: Portion Sizing Your Snacks

Ask family members to choose their favorite snack from the food that you currently have on hand at home and bring it to the kitchen table. Have them place the amount they usually consume on a plate or in a bowl. Each person should guess how much food (in cups) is in each plate or bowl. Then, using measuring cups, measure the amount for each food.

Read each food's nutrition label to answer the following questions:

1. What is the serving size?

2. How many servings are in 1 container?

3. How many calories are in 1 serving?

4. How many grams of added sugar are in 1 serving?

5. How many grams of fiber are in 1 serving?

6. How does your usual portion compare to a single portion size?

7. Considering the following nutrition targets, how healthy is your snack?
   - No more than 8 g of added sugar
   - No more than 10% of daily total calories
   - Two to 3 g of fiber
   - No more than 200 mg of sodium

❸ *Focus on fruits and vegetables.*

The best snacks are fruits and vegetables, and eating them is a great way to help kids meet the "5 a day" recommendation. Fruits and vegetables are full of fiber, which help kids feel full, along with many other nutrients, and they are free of added salt and sugar. If snacking only on fruits and vegetables will not work for your family, then at least try to limit snacks to 2 food groups, one of which is a vegetable or fruit. For snack ideas, check out the Your Toolbox: "Snacks Mix and Match" Box.

Your Toolbox: Snacks Mix and Match

Make snack time easier by letting kids create a healthy snack by choosing at least 1 vegetable or fruit to pair with either another vegetable or fruit or a whole grain or protein from the following list:

Vegetables	**Fruits**	**Whole Grains**	**Sample Snack Combinations**
Carrots	Apples	Whole wheat crackers	Apples and peanut butter
Celery	Bananas	Whole wheat bread	Celery sticks with peanut
Broccoli	Oranges	Whole wheat pita chips	butter and raisins or dried
Cucumbers	Strawberry	Pretzels	cranberries ("ants on a log")
Olives	Watermelon	Cheerios	Hummus with pretzels
Peppers	Apricot, peaches,		Frozen grapes
Tomatoes	nectarines	**Proteins**	Edamame
Jicama	Grapes, raisins	Peanut or sunflower butter	Hard-boiled egg and tomato
Seaweed	Berries	Nuts or seeds	slices
	Melon	Hard-boiled egg	Avocado toast
		Hummus	
		Edamame	

Sweets

We are all born with a preference for sweet foods, and kids especially tend to crave sweets and desserts. Help your kids lower their sugar intake by 'scheduling' desserts into your eating plan. Instead of including a dessert after most lunches and/or dinners, schedule desserts for specific days and meals. For example, agree ahead of time how many days per week you will have desserts and build them into your meal plan. The kids then can look forward to dessert days, but since they know the desserts "rule," they will learn to not beg for desserts every night. Make or purchase sweets and desserts as single portions to avoid having leftovers sitting around the house (because, of course, the kids will want to eat them!) (see KITCHEN HACKS "Portion Control Your Cookies" Box). This plan can help the adults in your house curb a sweet tooth as well.

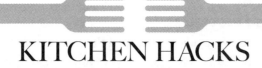

KITCHEN HACKS

Portion Control Your Cookies

The next time you make cookies (eg, the oatmeal banana chocolate chip cookies in the Appendix), make portion control easy by using parchment or wax paper on your cookie sheet. Drop the dough on the parchment or wax paper as if you are going to bake the cookies, but instead of putting the cookies in the oven, place the parchment or wax paper with the cookies on it in the freezer. Once the cookies are frozen, transfer them to a freezer bag. Then, when you want a cookie, take single-serving sizes of the cookies from the freezer and bake them.

However you choose to handle it, portion control is an important tool in helping your children rely on cues of hunger and fullness to decide how much to eat rather than the amount of food that's sitting in front of them.

Sugary Drinks

Whenever possible, it is better to eat your calories than drink them. Calories from food (especially minimally processed food) help increase the feeling of fullness much more than an equal number of calories from a drink. Because drinks don't cause fullness, people tend to eat the same amount of food as they otherwise would, regardless of how many calories they drink. This ends up leading to overeating and excess weight gain. Plus, most drinks contain a lot more sugar than you would think. And that extra sugar is associated with serious health consequences, such as obesity, diabetes, fatty liver disease, high blood pressure, heart disease, and tooth decay.

Whether plain, sparkling, or infused, water is the best drink for kids and adults. Milk and no-added-sugar milk substitutes also have an important role in helping meet calcium and vitamin D requirements, but most other types of drinks are best avoided or at least limited to fewer than one 8-ounce serving per week.

Note that even healthy-seeming drinks, such as 100% juice, toddler drinks, and green smoothies, contain sugar. Help your kids get an idea of how much sugar is lurking in their drinks with our sugary drink game in the LET'S EXPERIMENT "Sugary Drinks" Box.

LET'S EXPERIMENT: Sugary Drinks

Select a few sugary drinks that are family favorites (eg, juice, sports drink, soda, chocolate milk). Measure out the number of ounces that is equivalent to 1 serving. (Look at the drink's nutrition label to find this information.) Look for the number of grams of added sugar. Each 4 g of added sugars equals 1 teaspoon of sugar. There are 3 teaspoons in a tablespoon. In a sandwich bag or other container, measure out table sugar in the amount listed on the nutrition label.

Ask the kids to imagine that they are eating that amount of sugar every time they drink the sugary drink. Which drinks have the most sugar? Did anything surprise you? Ask the kids for some ideas of what might be a healthier drink. The following are a few key points you might make as you discuss this activity with your kids:

- Sugary drinks should be limited to no more than one 8-ounce serving per week, ideally fewer.
- The added-sugar goal for kids is no more than 25 g per day, and that amount includes both foods—many of which contain an abundance of added sugars—and drinks.
- Drinking sparkling water can be a helpful strategy to transition from soda.
- Zero-calorie drinks that are sweetened with nonnutritive sweeteners can help with the transition from full-sugar drinks; however, the goal is to eliminate sweet drinks altogether, especially for kids, because the long-term safety of nonnutritive sweeteners is a bit uncertain.

Screen Time

Because of the prevalence of smartphones, video games, computers, and television, most of us spend a lot more time in front of a screen than we spend with each other or being physically active. In fact, a study of teenagers found that although teens admit that they spend too much time with their devices, more than half also feel that their parents do as well. (For more on this study, as well as fast facts on teens, adults, and media use, check out the Did You Know? "Fast Facts: Teens, Parents, and Media Use" Box). It may be unrealistic to get rid of the screens. After all, being tech savvy is essential for success. But limiting screen time is a healthy practice. During week 3, focus on the screen time SMART goals and action plans you developed in preparation for the Family Fit Plan (see Chapter 3) or use the ones that I suggested. In addition, consider implementing the following screen time guidelines and watch how it transforms your family.

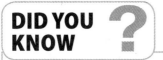

DID YOU KNOW

FAST FACTS: TEENS, PARENTS, AND MEDIA USE
- 95% of teens have access to a smartphone.
- 72% of teens say they often or sometimes check their phone as soon as they wake up.
- 97% of teen boys play video games.
- 85% of teens use YouTube, 72% use Instagram, and 69% use Snapchat. These are the 3 most popular social media platforms among teens.
- 45% of teens say they are online "almost constantly."
- 56% of teens feel anxious, lonely, or upset when they don't have their phone with them.
- 50% of teens are trying to limit their own screen time.
- 51% of teens say a parent is distracted by their own smartphone when a teen is trying to have a conversation, while 70% of parents say the same about their teens.
- 67% of parents are concerned their teen spends too much time on the phone.
- 36% of parents feel that they themselves spend too much time on their phone.
- 15% of parents say they lose focus at work because of their phone.
- 57% of parents set some type of screen restriction on their teens.

Sources: Jiang J. How teens and parents navigate screen time and device distractions. Pew Research Center website. http://www.pewinternet.org/ 2018/08/22/how-teens-and-parents-navigate-screen-time-and-device-distractions. Published August 22, 2018. Accessed March 18, 2019, and Anderson M, Jiang J. Teens, social media & technology 2018. Pew Research Center website. http://www.pewinternet.org/2018/05/31/teens-social-media-technology-2018. Published May 31, 2018. Accessed March 18, 2019

1. Schedule screen time.

Reduce screen time battles by making a schedule with clear rules for when screen time is allowed. For example, in response to behavior and attention concerns and continued battles, we set a clear rule for my school-aged kids that my husband and I consistently enforce: the kids are not allowed non–school-required screen time Monday through Thursday. On Fridays, the kids are allowed 1 hour of screen time, with some flexibility to watch a movie. On weekends, they are allowed up to 2 hours. We have a more difficult time enforcing the time cap on the weekends, but everyone knows the rules and we stick to it for the most part. Although it is more difficult to police teen screen time, you can work together with a teen to come up with a screen time schedule. Adults also benefit from imposing a schedule on themselves. If you find that you spend a lot of time on social media, for example, you might reclaim some of your time by allowing yourself a set amount of time at a set time of day or limit your number of check-ins per day.

2. Remove screens from bedrooms.

When kids and teens have screens in their bedrooms, they are more likely to spend more time in their rooms, away from other family members. In addition, they potentially may be exposed to media that is not appropriate for their age or beneficial to their mental health. The advice to remove screens from the bedroom also pertains to adults, if possible. Make it the norm to store smartphones and other devices overnight in the kitchen or living room. For adults who need to keep a cell phone close by overnight, take extra steps to make it easier to resist the temptation to read on the phone right before bed or picking up the phone when it is hard to fall asleep or get back to sleep after waking in the night.

3. Strict rule: no screen time (including smartphones) within 1 hour of going to bed.

The backlighting on TVs, smartphones, and computers can make it difficult to fall asleep. This rule will help make falling asleep easier for the whole family.

4. Strict rule: no screens allowed during mealtimes.

Use of devices during mealtimes is detrimental for at least 2 reasons. First, it sets up mindless eating, as we tend to eat more and enjoy the food less when we are distracted. Secondly, it detracts from the opportunity to spend time connecting and socializing with the rest of the family.

The American Academy of Pediatrics (AAP) Family Media Use Plan can help you put into practice these rules and others that your family agrees on. The AAP Family Media Use Plan also offers guidance on choosing quality and age-appropriate media during recreational screen time, media manners, and digital citizenship. If you haven't already done so, create your family's plan at www.HealthyChildren.org/mediauseplan. If you have already included components of your own Family Media Use Plan in your SMART goals and action steps for the Family Fit Plan, now is a good time to check in on how it has been going and make updates to your plan.

Sleep Disruptors

Poor sleep wreaks havoc on a family. Not only does it decrease patience, but it also is associated with overeating, decreased physical activity, and poor general health. In preparation for the Family Fit Plan, you likely developed SMART goals and action steps to help improve sleep (see Chapter 3). Similar to week 3's focus on your screen time goals, it's also a great time to evaluate progress toward your sleep goals. It may help to try to identify and resolve sleep disruptors. The following are common causes of poor sleep and what to do about them:

- **Lack of healthy sleep routines.** Kids fall asleep and stay asleep more easily if they follow a consistent bedtime routine. If you haven't already done so, try implementing the 5 Bs described in week 2.
- **Screen time too close to bedtime** or using the screen (eg, TV, movies, browsing the internet) to fall asleep. Keep screens out of bedrooms and enforce a rule of no screen time within 1 hour of bedtime.
- **Nighttime waking.** Use the mindful breathing described in week 2 to help you fall back to sleep after waking in the night. Teach your kids to do the same.
- **Poorly timed caffeine intake** for adults or any caffeine intake for kids. Avoid drinking anything with caffeine too late in the day. The caffeine can make it more difficult to fall asleep and can also cause nighttime waking.
- **Depression.** People who have depression tend to sleep either much more than is normal for them or much less. If you are concerned you or a family member may have depression, seek help from your physician or a local mental health professional. Psychologytoday.com offers a search option to help find a licensed psychologist near you.
- **Snoring and sleep apnea.** Snoring disrupts the quality of sleep for both the person who snores and those who hear the snoring as they try to sleep. If you or a family member snores, and especially if there are any pauses in breathing during snoring, see a doctor for evaluation and possible treatment.

Slick Sales and Marketing

Kids' opinions about most things, including foods to eat, can be heavily influenced by savvy sales and marketing tactics. The food industry has particularly deep pockets and skilled marketing professionals who know how to appeal to their target audience. Although there are rules in place to protect children from sophisticated marketing campaigns, the reality is that children are bombarded with food and beverage ads, mostly promoting unhealthful choices. In an editorial published several years ago in the *New England Journal of Medicine*, Marion Nestle, an outspoken nutrition advocate and professor of nutrition at New York University, described the underlying agenda of food marketers to build brand loyalty by teaching children brand recognition, encouraging kids to pester their parents to buy the advertised products, and convincing children they need special foods made just for them.

The strategy works. Children who spend 30 minutes or more per day online are twice as likely to pester their parents for junk food than kids who stay off-line. By 2 years of age, kids are able to recognize advertised products at supermarkets and ask for them by name. And many children routinely report that they—not their parents—decide what they eat. Kids exposed to the advertisements consistently request and choose advertised foods more often and report liking the foods better than their peers who did not see the ads. Because most foods advertised are high in sugar, calories, or sodium, television and online viewing directly impedes your efforts to have your kids eat better. In fact, kids who spend 3 or more hours per day online are 4 times more likely to buy junk food and 80% more likely to have overweight or obesity. They also are at increased risk for 13 types of cancers compared with kids with screen limits.

Screen time also gets in the way of your ability to raise your children in a peaceful environment. When your child begs you to purchase a product seen advertised and you say "no," your child is very likely to become disappointed or upset. In fact, a research review found a significant relationship between a child's advertising exposure, materialism, and parent-child conflict. Even if you limit exposure to TV and online advertisements, children see food advertisements elsewhere (eg, at school, on billboards, in movies, with friends). Two important strategies work hand in hand to help dull the influence of sales and marketing on your kids' behaviors: limit their exposure and teach them media literacy.

Limit Exposure

As food marketers have become more sophisticated, product placement pops up everywhere, including on websites, apps, social media, movies, songs, toys, games, educational materials, text messages, celebrity endorsements, and even celebrity tweets. While you cannot completely protect your child from exposure to advertisements, you can limit it. If your younger kids will be watching television, choose stations such as PBS Kids where commercials are not allowed, or record a program on a DVR and fast-forward through the commercials when viewing. Be mindful of what your kids are doing and seeing online. Restrict games and apps that include in-app advertisements. Shop at grocery stores where food packaging tends to be plain and does not have brightly colored cartoonish front-of-package labeling that tries to appeal to children. Or strategically shop at the grocery store to decrease exposure to the battle-inducing heavily advertised candies and snacks (ie, shop the perimeter, which is mostly produce and fresh food, and avoid candy and chip aisles). If exposure cannot be avoided, hold firm when refusing to purchase the heavily advertised junk foods that your child so adamantly insists on buying.

Teach Media Literacy

Recognizing the role of food marketing in dictating your child's food requests and preferences is the first step in defending against its influence. In the long run, teaching your kids to be savvy consumers is the most effective strategy to limit the negative effect of food marketing, especially for kids aged 7 years and older. (Kids younger than 7 years usually do not have the cognitive ability to discern commercials from programming.) Media literacy is especially important to teach your teens, as they are key targets of junk food and soda advertisements. Follow these 3 ways to teach your kids media literacy:

Teach Your Kids to Be Critical of Advertisements

The foundation of media literacy training is to teach children to be critical of advertisements. To do that, explain to your kids that the purpose of an advertisement is to get you to buy something. The advertiser's goal is to persuade you to want what it is selling. While they are not allowed to lie, they can exaggerate. They are biased. Biased messages should be taken with a grain of salt.

Teach Your Kids That Advertisers Use Several Tried-and-true Strategies to Persuade

An overview of a few of the mostly commonly used strategies follows:

Celebrity appeal. A clear marketing strategy to lure teens to choose advertised products is to attach celebrity endorsements to those products. In fact, a 2016 study found that junk foods were a key product promoted by top celebrities. At that time, 65 celebrities (most of whom had a Teen Choice Award nomination) were collectively associated with 57 different food and beverage brands, of which more than 70% of promoted drinks were sugary drinks and 80% of foods were junk food. Another study looked at how social media influencers (like teenaged YouTube stars) affect viewers' food intake. While endorsement by the YouTube "celebrities" increased junk food intake among viewers, it had little effect on intake of healthy foods like fruits and vegetables.

Licensed characters. Putting the faces of licensed characters, such as Pokémon, SpongeBob SquarePants, Paw Patrol, My Little Pony, and various other popular children's icons, on products is a surefire way to sell them. In one study, children tasted cereal from a plain box and the same cereal with the penguins Mumble and Gloria from *Happy Feet* on the box. The kids said they liked the cereal from the penguin-adorned box more, even though it was the exact same cereal. You can attempt this strategy at home to promote healthier habits. Help younger kids see that their cartoon friends also like healthy foods. Decorate a snack bag with Paw Patrol stickers and see if that helps to increase the appeal of the edamame you've offered your toddler for a snack. Or help your teen see how some favorite artists healthfully incorporate fitness into their lives.

Emotional appeal. An important component of a successful marketing campaign is to create an emotional experience.

- **Excitement.** The marketers want kids to believe this product is the key to amazing fun and adventure. One sip and you're dancing onstage with Taylor Swift. You can create excitement by serving snacks with fun plates, napkins, cups, or straws or having a tasting party where children can vote for their favorite healthy snacks.
- **Feel good.** This type of ad tells a story that makes you feel good. For example, a dad cheers up his daughter by taking her to lunch at their favorite fast-food chain. This strategy is used by the McDonald's Corporation with its "Happy Meal," which also throws in an enticing toy for added appeal. This method of advertising is so effective that Coca-Cola made its tagline "Taste the feeling" and rolled out a series of ads showing images of friends and families connecting over a soda. Try this strategy by packaging favorite family activities with memories of healthy food offerings. For example, a family picnic reunion might always include cutting up a watermelon and having seed-spitting contests.
- **Sounds good.** Ads often include music to catch your attention, and when they are most effective, they can stay with you for decades. Children of the 1980s may still be able to sing the jingle or associate the brand with any of these songs used in commercials: "Give me a break. Give me a break. Break me off a piece of that…," or "I'm lovin' it." Make up fun songs to sing about your child's favorite healthy foods. For example, *Sesame Street* aired the catchy song and character "Captain Vegetable," who sings about his love of vegetables.

Repetition. Manufacturers hope that if you see a product or hear its name over and over again, you'll want it. Sometimes, the same ad is repeated several times during a 1-hour television broadcast. Frequently offer the foods you want your kids to love. Prepare them in different ways, but continue to offer them. Remember, it takes 15 times or more for a child to accept a previously rejected food.

Packaging. Putting nutrition claims on packaged products is good business for food manufacturers. It increases the perceived healthfulness of the food, which translates into increased sales. Manufacturers frequently mislead consumers by highlighting the content of single ingredients that are associated with health, such as vitamins A, C, and D; calcium; fiber; and omega 3s. They also promote "organic" and "gluten-free" labels. But don't fall for it—just because a fruit snack lists that it has "100% of vitamin C" doesn't mean it's healthy. Likewise, a food that lists itself as being organic or gluten free doesn't necessarily make it healthier. For example, any of these foods could still be, and often are, loaded with sugar.

The Prevention Institute conducted a study to see whether front-of-package labels on "better-for-you" foods marketed to kids actually promoted foods that were healthy. It turns out that 84% of the foods were considered unhealthy based on their saturated fat, sugar, sodium, or (lack of) fiber content. In addition, the researchers also found that 13% of beverages, 40% of cereals, and 50% of snack foods contained food dye additives to make foods more brightly colored and thus more appealing to kids. Artificial coloring has been linked to hyperactivity, allergic reactions, and other harmful outcomes in kids. The coloring often is used to simulate fruits, but, as an earlier Prevention Institute study showed, despite clear references to fruits on product packaging, nearly two-thirds of the most heavily advertised foods targeting kids contained little or no fruit at all. The unfortunate reality is that it's very difficult to find processed foods that are nutritious, despite what the food manufacturers would like you to think.

Practice

After you have helped your kids identify the strategies that marketers often use, keep a lookout for advertisements everywhere—on TV, online, in apps, on billboards, at the movies, and on buses. Then, together with your child, analyze them. Identify what strategies the advertisers use to try to persuade you. Are they compelling? What's the actual nutritional value of the product? What healthier and less expensive alternatives that taste just as good could you try instead?

Family Meeting: Outsmarting the 6 Ss

During week 3, take note if any common barriers (eg, the 6 Ss) may be getting in the way of achieving your goals.

✔ Open the meeting by reviewing your nutrition, sleep, and screen time goals and action steps.

✔ Share that week 3's focus is on common barriers that can make it harder to reach our health goals. Ask family members to share if they can think of any barriers that has made making changes harder. Note if any of the 6 Ss are mentioned (snacks, sweets, sugary drinks, screen time, sleep disruptors, slick sales).

✔ **Activity:** Choose 1 of the following activities to do during your family meeting:
  - Play the "size your snacks" game.
  - Play the "sugary drinks" game.
  - Develop a Family Media Use Plan if you haven't already. If you already have a plan, check in on how well your family is following it.
  - Discuss media literacy, and watch 10 minutes of your kids' favorite online game or show and track the advertisements you see, including the venue, type of advertisement, and products advertised.

✔ **Activity for the week:** Make plans to incorporate as many of the following Activities for the Week as you reasonably can:
  - Self-monitor nutrition, physical activity, screen time, and sleep using the Family Fit Tracker (see Appendix).
  - Map out your weekly meal plan (see the Weekly Meal Planner and recipe ideas in the Appendix).
  - Map out your weekly fitness plan (see the Family Fit Tracker in the Appendix).
  - Map out and post your family schedule.
  - Create and enforce a schedule around snacks, sleep, and screen time.
  - Do any of the activities from the list above that you didn't have time to do during your family meeting.

✔ **Closing family activity:** Close week 3's meeting by asking each family member to share which of the 6 Ss each one would most like to focus on addressing this week.

Week 4: Savoring and Celebrating Success

The transition from infancy to toddlerhood is marked by extraordinary developmental advances. Perhaps the most iconic is that of the 12-month-old who bravely stands alone, fearful, attempting to take a first step. The baby's parents are sitting on the ground, arms out, smiles on their faces. She falls. They applaud her effort and root for her to try again. She gets up. And she falls. With a determined look on her face, she gets up again and successfully takes a step. Her parents applaud and cheer. She starts clapping for herself before she sits down, beaming. This experience of a child taking his or her first step is a memory that most parents hold dear. Despite many failed attempts for their child to walk, parents encourage them, remain optimistic, and applaud the process and the resilience of a child who falls down only to get back up again. The experience is positive for everyone. The parents are quick to praise. They withhold criticism, recognizing their baby is learning a new skill, which takes time, patience, and developmental readiness.

But then, it is not too much later in a young toddler's development when he or she starts to say more words. Soon "no" enters the vocabulary. Parents ask their toddler to do something, and their toddler says "no." Curious, their toddler begins to explore new places around the house. Everywhere their toddler goes, worried for his or her safety, the parents say "no." As a toddler pushes the limits, parents push back. Whether it is potty training, eating, bedtime, or play, many toddlers come to challenge their parents' authority, setting up a battle of the wills. And most parents acknowledge that getting into a battle of the wills with a toddler is a surefire way to lose, with everyone leaving the experience in tears of frustration.

Early on in parenting, we are quick to praise our kids and their progress. But as time goes on— and we become increasingly sleep deprived, busy, and stressed—our tolerance decreases and, as is human nature, we spend more time and energy focused on "righting" what is wrong than recognizing and praising what is good. "Bad is stronger than good," wrote social psychologist Roy Baumeister and his colleagues in a journal article that explains the psychological phenomenon that "bad emotions, bad parents, and bad feedback have more impact than good ones."

It is human to pay more attention to setbacks and areas where things are not going well than to direct attention to what is going right and to our and our children's successes. We more deeply experience painful experiences than joyful ones. We are quicker to criticize mistakes and failures than to praise and celebrate successes. But "good can overcome bad by force of numbers. To maximize the power of good, these numbers must be increased.... Individuals can make an effort to recognize and appreciate the goods they have—celebrating each small success, being thankful for health, and having gratitude for supportive others." In fact, research suggests for "good to become stronger than bad," we need 5 positive experiences for every 1 negative.

Week 4's focus is on helping the good in your family's change plan overwhelm the bad by savoring and celebrating positive experiences. This approach also helps boost health in and of itself. For example, in their book, *Savoring,* social psychologists Fred Bryant and Joseph Veroff make a strong case for the health benefits of "being mindfully engaged and aware during positive events." This mindful engagement increases happiness, strengthens relationships, improves mental and physical health, and improves creativity. Bryant and Veroff describe 9 strategies to help savor positive experiences: *behavioral expression (celebrate), self-congratulations, sharing with others, memory building, temporal awareness ("slow down time"), counting your blessings, absorption, sensory-perceptual sharpening ("sharpen your senses"), and comparing.*

Over the course of week 4, you will practice ways to apply each of the strategies in your daily family routines. The outcome will be more profound and lasting positive experiences and a fun and rewarding final week of your Family Fit Plan. While you may find that certain savoring strategies come more naturally to you than others, take this week to experiment with each of these strategies. Hopefully you will find an approach that works best for you to savor and celebrate your and your family's successes.

Celebrate

Start the week by making a concerted effort to celebrate your family's successes, even the smallest ones. Finished the walk you had planned but didn't feel motivated to do? Fist bump! Made dinner after a hurried day when you really felt like going through the drive-through instead? "You rock!" Crossed another action plan off your list in pursuit of a SMART goal? Family dance party! While your family is working to achieve its goals, recognize the smallest successes and celebrate them in small ways. Perhaps it is a fitness gain, a recipe that turned out just right, or a child who helped clean up the dishes without being asked. Give high fives all around, pump your fist and say "yes!" or come up with your own special form of celebrating the small stuff. Start a running list of *all* your family's successes this week. Encourage everyone to add to it. Then have a plan for how to celebrate in a bigger way at the end of the week. Celebrations are inherently positive experiences that help to reward and reinforce continuing a positive behavior.

Figure 7.1. Sample Ways of Savoring Checklist
How do you savor positive experiences? Think of positive experiences you have had in the past. Check the "Did you do this?" box next to the statements that best describe how you responded to these types of experiences.

Example	Strategy	Did you do this?
I jumped up and down, ran around, or showed other physical expressions of energy.	Behavioral expression (celebrate)	
I told myself how proud I was.	Self-congratulations	
I thought about sharing the memory of this later with other people.	Sharing with others	
I thought about how I'd think to myself about this event later.	Memory building	
I reminded myself that it would be over before I knew it.	Temporal awareness ("Slow down time")	
I reminded myself how lucky I was to have this good thing happen to me.	Count your blessings	
I closed my eyes, relaxed, and took in the moment.	Absorption	
I opened my eyes wide, took a deep breath, and tried to become more alert.	Sensory-perceptual sharpening ("sharpen your senses")	
I thought back to events that led up to this experience—to a time when I didn't have it and wanted it.	Comparing	

Source: Used with permission from Bryant FB, Veroff J. *Savoring: A New Model of Positive Experience.* Mahwah, NJ: Lawrence Erlbaum Associates; 2007.

Pat Yourself on the Back

As you make celebrating successes a priority, don't forget to pause and offer yourself some self-congratulations. If you've completed your action plan, or accomplished a goal, reward yourself. Teach your children how to congratulate and reward themselves for succeeding and achieving their goals, without bragging or putting other people down. For example, perhaps they have a personal "brag journal" or they save their allowance to purchase a book or toy once they've reached a goal.

Share Your Positive Experiences With Each Other

Sharing a positive experience with another person helps to imprint the memory and strengthens the relationship with that person, furthering social support. Let your family know when you've completed your action steps or achieved a goal. And encourage them to share their positive experiences with you. You can build this into your weekly routine during your family dinners.

Go around the table and ask each person to share a positive experience or a recent accomplishment. Ask what he or she had to do to achieve that success. Help your kids associate hard work and follow-through with goal attainment.

Make New Memories Together

Creating a mental picture of a positive experience helps that moment live on in your memory and brings back positive emotions when you reminisce. By engaging many of your senses in the experience, a smell or sound can recreate those feelings far into the future. For example, do any songs from your childhood bring you back to a specific time from your past?

Build a new memory with your child during week 4 that you want both of you to hold on to forever. While the memory does not need to be elaborate, we tend to remember first experiences. Perhaps you could try a new activity neither of you have done before, such as trying out a new sport, ice skating or climbing a rock wall? Other activities like making a meal, taking a walk, going for a bike ride, gardening, or taking a yoga class together can create lasting memories, especially if during the activity you take in the surrounding sights, sounds, touches, tastes, and smells. For example, you might engage all your senses and create a memorable experience at home by lighting an aromatic candle and playing soft music while you complete a sun salutation beginner-yoga sequence together (see the GET FIT! "Yoga Sun Salutations for Beginners" Box). Once you have the experience, ask yourself what you want to remember the most. Then take a moment to reminisce on that part of the experience to help further imprint it into your memory. This type of special time also is a great reward for a child who has accomplished a goal or otherwise earned a reward.

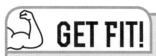 **GET FIT!** **YOGA SUN SALUTATIONS FOR BEGINNERS**

Create a lasting memory with your child while getting fit by completing the yoga sun salutations sequence for beginners. Engage all of your senses by playing soft music, lighting an aromatic candle, and taking deep mindful breaths while you go through the sequence shown in the Appendix.

Slow Down Time

Every new parent has heard a parent with older kids remark with some variation of "Enjoy them now—time flies" or "The days are long, but the years are short." Savoring life's big moments—births, birthdays, graduations, weddings—helps us hold the memories closer and brings joy in reminiscing. Our perception of time passing is tied closely with experiences. The stronger the emotion associated with the experience, for better or for worse, the longer the memory persists. During week 4, help slow down time by creating a new and salient experience with your kids. Try a new activity together for the first time, prepare a new food, or start a new tradition.

Count Your Blessings

Ralph Waldo Emerson said, "Cultivate the habit of being grateful for every good thing that comes to you, and to give thanks continuously. And because all things have contributed to your advancement, you should include all things in your gratitude." Regularly expressing gratitude is associated with happiness, kindness, health, and well-being. Grateful teens are happier, more optimistic, better supported, and more satisfied with their relationships at home and school and with friends. They also tend to be more engaged in their schoolwork and hobbies, have better grades, and are less susceptible to envy and depression. Add gratitude practice to your Family Fit Plan to help the whole family get in the habit of giving thanks and showing genuine appreciation. The following suggestions are a few ways you can get started:

✔ At the beginning of mealtimes, go around the table and ask each person to say 1 thing that he or she is thankful for that day. To add variety, you could ask questions such as
  - "Who made you smile today?"
  - "Who helped you solve a tough problem today?"
  - "Who made you feel better when you had a tough day?"
  - "What made you feel good today?"

✔ Model good manners while also reminding children to use good manners, saying things like "please," "thank you," and "excuse me." Give them many opportunities to practice, including ordering their own food when you go out to restaurants.

✔ Model gratitude with genuine compliments and expressions of appreciation with other family members. For example, say things like, "I appreciate that you were willing to try the new food," or "Thank you for going on the walk with me. It meant a lot to me to be able to spend that time with you." In addition to verbal appreciation, consider written appreciation as well. For example, leave a sticky note for each family member stating something you appreciate.

✔ Write a gratitude letter. Help the kids write a letter of gratitude to someone to whom they would like to thank or show appreciation.

✔ Count blessings each night before you go to sleep. Help kids get into a routine of adding appreciation to their bedtime routine. This can be part of a bedtime meditation as they are falling asleep in which they think of 3 good things that happened that day. Older kids and adults might consider keeping a gratitude journal in which they think of and write down 3 good things that happened each day and reflect on why they happened.

Absorb Yourself in the Moment

Have you ever had an experience in which you were so focused on doing something that you were lost in the moment, without sense of time or place? You may have been experiencing *flow state*. This experience, first described by psychologist Mihaly Csikszentmihalyi, occurs when a person is so deeply absorbed in a challenging, intrinsically motivating activity that he or she loses a sense of time and place. A person in flow is free of self-consciousness and experiences goal clarity, complete concentration, feelings of control, and being completely absorbed in the activity. This is the state elite athletes aspire to, the experience when peak performance occurs. But flow is not limited to elite athletes. It can be experienced by anyone. Spending time in flow helps to improve happiness, positive affect, and performance and behavior. You may have experienced flow in the past if you can respond positively to the following situations:

- I was challenged, but I believed my skills would allow me to meet the challenge.
- My attention was focused entirely on what I was doing.
- Time seemed to alter (either slowed down or sped up).
- Things just seemed to be happening automatically.
- It was no effort to keep my mind on what was happening.
- I was not worried about what others may have been thinking of me.
- I found the experience extremely rewarding.

Studies have found that adolescents who experience flow have improved concentration, happiness, strength, self-esteem, optimism, and intrinsic motivation. Teens who grow up in families with a high degree of support, harmony, involvement, and freedom are more likely to experience flow. They also report a more positive home environment, happiness, sociability, motivation, self-esteem, and a sense of living up to their own and others' expectations. A teen's "yes" answers to most or all of the questions in the Your Toolbox: "Do You Have a 'Complex' Family?" Box are reflective of these types of families.

During week 4, try to create opportunities for flow experiences. The best activities are those in which skill level and challenge both are high, but this is not always necessary. For example, a walk in the woods, a long bike ride, mindful meditation, a run, gardening, cooking, playing music, dancing, making art, or creative play all can offer flow opportunities.

Sharpen Your Senses

Our 5 senses of sight, sound, taste, touch, and smell help us to fully experience the world. The taste of a decadent meal. The sound of a newborn's cry. The touch of a friend's embrace. The smell of a rose or the beauty of a piece of art. Often, the stimuli are too much for our brain to process all at once, so we attend to that which is most dominant or pressing. In the hurriedness

Your Toolbox: Do You Have a "Complex" Family?

A teen's "yes" answers to most or all of the following questions suggest a "complex" family, characterized by high support, harmony, involvement, and freedom. These questions are derived from the Complex Family Questionnaire:

- Are there objects around the house (eg, photos, paintings, heirlooms, prized possessions) that hold special memories for family members?

- Are other family members serious and intense when engaging with things that are important to them?

- Are there clear rules that keep the house running smoothly?

- If you are feeling depressed or are having a problem, do others notice even though you may not say anything about it?

- Can you find a place to find privacy and to escape into your own world at home when you need to?

- Would you say your family is religious or spiritual, even though they may not attend church regularly?

- Does your family have traditional ways of celebrating birthdays that enhance a feeling of family togetherness and unity?

- Do other family members modify their plans on your behalf (ie, are you sometimes the center of attention)?

- Are members of your family consistent in their actions?

- Is there a strong competitive spirit at home when family members play games or sports?

- Are family members proud, do they work hard, and do they have ideals and values?

If your teen is willing, discuss the questions to which your teen answered "no" and explore what changes, if any, are in order to help increase your family's "complexity."

Source: Used with permission from Csikszentmihalyi M, Rathune K, Whalen S. *Talented Teenagers: The Roots of Success and Failure*. Cambridge: Cambridge University Press; 1997.

of raising a family, balancing multiple schedules, and sleep deprivation, we often are left with limited reserve at the end of the day to savor the good moments. But if we take the time to pay attention to our senses, we can come to see the world, and our daily experiences, in a different way. You may see your kids every day, but when was the last time you focused all of your attention, free of distraction of activity or thought, to observe them play? When did you last listen to the sound of a child's breathing while drifting off to sleep? Have you noticed how closing your eyes before tasting a food can enhance its flavor? Increase your appreciation of everyday beauty and sharpen your senses by taking a savoring walk in which you notice all of the positive things you can, including sights, sounds, and smells. Make a concerted effort to experience and savor your food with the activity in the Mindful Moment: "Savor Your Food Activity" Box.

Mindful Moment: Savor Your Food Activity

Follow these 7 steps to sharpen your senses as you savor your food:

1. Ensure the room is completely quiet.

2. Observe your food. Notice the nooks and crannies and observe the food's texture.

3. Smell the food by bringing your nose close to the food and inhaling deeply through your nose.

4. Feel the texture of the food in your mouth as you take a small bite.

5. Taste the blend of flavors on your tongue.

6. Chew the food slowly.

7. Swallow.

Sharpening Your Child's Sense of Taste

Honing the 5 senses not only can help you savor and appreciate the small miracles all around you, but it also can help you make progress in your Family Fit Plan and goal of raising healthier kids with more adventurous taste preferences. Although taste is the strongest predictor of whether a child will eat a food, a child forms an opinion of whether or not something will taste good by how it looks and smells. How many times have you heard children say they don't like a food that they've never actually tasted? Once a child chooses to taste the food, the taste and texture (touch) of the food influence the child's perception of liking the food or not.

Babies exposed to a wide variety of healthy foods (first in utero through amniotic fluid, next through maternal breast milk, and then in the first several months of exposure to solid foods) generally like a wide variety of foods. Have you ever wondered why most kids in India or Thailand love curry while many children raised in the United States balk at even the faintest hint of spice? If you expose your children to a wide variety of food tastes from a young age, you'll raise kids with not only a more sophisticated palate but also a higher tolerance for trying new foods.

A child doesn't need to chew and swallow a food to experience the food's taste. Even touching the food with the tongue allows a child to taste a food. The sense of taste comes from what are known as papillae, or little bumps on the outside border of the tongue. These papillae house taste buds that allow us to experience 5 different types of taste: sweet, sour, bitter, salty, and umami. Umami is derived from a Japanese word meaning "delicious" or "savory." Umami occurs naturally in many vegetables, such as mushrooms and tomatoes. It's also found in foods that are aged, including soy sauce, cheeses, and fermented products. For a taste of umami, check out the Grilled Portabella Mushroom Burger (With Sun-dried Tomato Yogurt Aioli) recipe in the Appendix.

The taste buds at the tip of the tongue are more sensitive to sour, while those at the back of the tongue are more sensitive to bitter. We are born liking the taste of sweet and salty foods, but most people have to learn to like bitter, sour, and umami through repeated exposures. A child being willing to try a food by putting it in his or her mouth and then spitting it out can help "train the taste buds" to eventually enjoy the food.

Individual foods can be enhanced with the addition of seasonings, spices, herbs, and seeds.

Seasonings are ingredients added to food that enhance the food's flavor without being specifically tasted themselves. Salt and pepper are basic seasonings that improve the flavor of a food. Although salt adds flavor, it also contributes to high blood pressure for some people. Thus, it's best to use minimal amounts of salt. Both black and white ground pepper add flavor to dark-colored foods without any increased risk of negative health effects; however, pepper may spoil the appearance of light-colored foods.

Herbs and spices add flavor to meals. Try these vegetable, herb, and spice combinations that often are used in cooking foods from different regions and countries.

- Indian: garlic + onion + curry powder + cinnamon
- Asian: garlic + scallions + sesame + ginger + soy sauce
- Italian: garlic + basil + parsley + oregano
- Middle Eastern: garlic + onion + mint + cumin + saffron + lemon
- Mexican: cumin + onion + oregano + cilantro

Some recipe ideas with these combinations are included in the Appendix. When you try them out, consider making your meal part of a cultural experience. For example, you could take your kids on a pretend trip around the world by learning about various countries and then preparing traditional meals from some of those places.

When a sweet, sour, bitter, or salty substance touches the tongue, a message is rapidly sent to the brain to help identify the taste. At the same time the brain is processing a food's taste, it's getting another message from the smell center in the nose. The sense of smell is powerful—it can differentiate hundreds of distinct odors. That makes it 10,000 times more sensitive than the sense of taste. Simply smelling a delicious food or a familiar scent can rapidly bring back memories of another time, when you smelled that food (eg, a whiff of fresh-baked cookies might immediately bring you back to when you were a child visiting Grandma's house). This is the perfect example of the intersection between food and eating, and how sometimes people may eat for reasons other than hunger, such as to bring back fond childhood memories. Of course, you can also use this to your advantage. If your children's meals smell and taste good, they'll prefer those tempting smells and delicious flavors when they're older. Pair this with a pleasant experience at family mealtimes and your kids are likely to remember and reproduce these experiences when they are older with their own families.

Texture, temperature, color, and shape also affect whether a child likes a food. Texture includes the qualities you can feel with your fingers, tongue, palate, or teeth. Almost everyone likes crispy, crunchy, tender, juicy, and firm textures. Most people dislike tough, soggy, crumbly, lumpy, watery, and slimy textures. Keep this in mind when preparing your meals. For example, when steaming vegetables, err on the side of not cooking enough (leaving a little bit of crunch) rather than cooking too much (leading to soggy). Check out the KITCHEN HACKS "Roasting Veggies and Ripening Fruits" Box for tips to make your vegetables and fruits taste delicious.

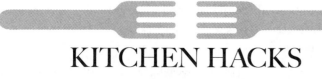

KITCHEN HACKS

Roasting Veggies and Ripening Fruits

Rely on roasted vegetables to help your family boost vegetable intake. They are easy to prepare and cook, and they taste delicious. Make your roasted vegetables taste even better by preheating your baking sheet. This enhances flavor and makes for even browning. Simply turn the oven on, put your pan in the oven, cut up and season your vegetables, take out the pan, add the vegetables, and bake. (See the roasted vegetables recipe in the Appendix.)

Perfectly and quickly ripen fruits by placing them in a paper lunch bag and fold the top to close. Fruit ripens by releasing a gas. The bag traps this gas, causing the fruit to ripen more quickly. Store the bag in a cool dry place out of direct sunlight for a day or 2 and voila, you have perfectly ripened and delicious fruit. This works especially well for peaches, pears, avocadoes, mangos, and tomatoes. Bananas and apples release extra amounts of ripening gas, so if you need your fruit soft in a hurry, add a banana or apple to the bag.

Temperature affects how tastes are experienced. The same amount of sugar tastes sweeter at higher temperatures, while the opposite is true for salt—the same amount of salt tastes saltier at lower temperatures. For the best flavor (and best chances your child will eat them), serve foods at their ideal temperature. Also, if you combine cold and hot temperatures in the same dish (eg, mango salsa on baked mahi-mahi) or mix hot and spicy foods, your food will be more flavorful.

A food's appearance can determine whether a kid is interested in giving it a try or rejects it outright. As you plan meals, rather than choosing bland-appearing but balanced meals, try to incorporate a variety of different colors. This will make the meal more appealing, and because fruits and vegetables are the most colorful foods, it ensures that you have ample fruits and vegetables containing a balanced mix of nutrients. For example, a meal of wild rice, tomato and basil chicken, red grapes, roasted sweet potatoes, and milk is more visually appealing than brown rice, grilled chicken, applesauce, roasted potatoes, and milk. The shape of food can also affect whether a child is willing to give it a try. For example, Mickey Mouse whole wheat pancakes are going to be a much bigger hit with the kids than the standard circular kind. A heart-shaped turkey sandwich holds much more appeal than a cut-down-the-middle sandwich.

Enhance the Senses by Age and Stage

Help your kids use their senses to prefer a wider variety of foods by following these strategies.

Infant (0–1 Year)

The sense of taste in infancy is very poorly developed and non-discriminating. That is, you can get an infant to try just about anything. Breastfeeding mothers can take advantage of this by eating a varied diet that includes many different flavors. This early exposure to many tastes helps prevent picky eating later. Once solids are introduced at around 6 months, gradually introduce an increasing variety and quality of flavors. This way, when your child develops neophobia (the fear of trying new foods) at around 2 years, not all that many flavors will be new.

Toddler (1–3 Years)

The toddler years are the toughest when it comes to getting the average kid to be willing to try—much less like—healthy foods. Everyone knows of a toddler who gets into a macaroni-and-cheese or peanut-butter-and-jelly rut. Remember, toddlers like tastes that are familiar to them. Bridge familiar tastes to newer tastes and textures by slightly modifying a mealtime favorite. For example, help a child who loves French fries come to like healthier vegetables by switching to sweet potato fries and then green bean fries. You can find recipes for both dishes in the Appendix.

Preschooler (3–5 Years)

The presentation and visual appeal of meals and snacks take center stage in the preschool years. Presenting food in cool shapes, multiple colors, and adornments entices a preschooler to give it a try. If you also make sure it tastes good, you're likely to have long-term success in raising a child who prefers the healthy foods. If you don't already own them, borrow the books *Green Eggs and Ham* by Dr Seuss (New York: Random House; 1960) and *The Very Hungry Caterpillar* by Eric Carle (New York: World Publishing Company; 1969) from the library and read them with your preschooler or toddler. You'll notice that these books relate well to the past few weeks of your Family Fit Plan.

School Age (5–11 Years)

By now, your child's taste preferences are fairly well established. This is great news if you have an adventurous eater who loves fruits and vegetables and is willing to try new tastes and textures, even if they are bitter or spicy. However, if your child prefers greasy or highly processed foods and shuns vegetables, fruits, and other healthful foods, then you have a little more work to do. To transition this child to preferring a wholesome fruit and veggie–rich diet, you'll have to make sure the food you're making tastes great. Instead of adding a lot of salt, sugar, or fat, consider experimenting with seasonings and herbs to give an old taste a new flare. Consider reading and discussing the book *The Ugly Vegetables* by Grace Lin (Watertown, MA: Charlesbridge; 2001) with your child.

Adolescent (12+ Years)

Adolescents are known for loving not-so-healthy foods like sodas and hot chips, but they also tend to be more willing to try new and different foods. A great way to get your teens to try new foods is to have them join you in the kitchen in preparing recipes. Ask your teen to choose an interesting recipe that you can make together (see Appendix). Or perhaps there is a local cooking class your teen would like to take.

Compare

The last of the savoring strategies to test during week 4 is comparing. How is your life today better than in the past, or how would it have been if you hadn't made certain positive life-changing choices? Take time to reflect on how your choices have helped your life turn out for the better. In the short term, compare your life today to what it was before you started the Family

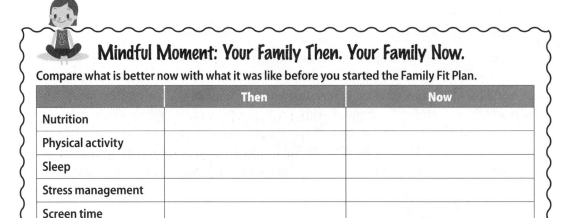

Mindful Moment: Your Family Then. Your Family Now.

Compare what is better now with what it was like before you started the Family Fit Plan.

	Then	Now
Nutrition		
Physical activity		
Sleep		
Stress management		
Screen time		

Fit Plan. What is better? What makes you the proudest? What could have been a consequence if you didn't make a change? The Mindful Moment: "Your Family Then. Your Family Now." Box helps you fill in the pieces to see how the small steps you've taken in the past few weeks have added up.

Family Meeting: Savoring and Celebrating Success

During week 4, practice savoring and celebrating.

✔ Open the meeting by making a list of each family member's favorite way to celebrate. Decide on how you would like to celebrate completing the Family Fit Plan at the end of this week.

✔ **Activity:** Choose one of the following activities to do during your family meeting:

- Complete the "Savor Your Food" activity (see Mindful Moment: "Savor Your Food Activity" Box).
- Write a gratitude letter.
- Ask everyone to share something great that happened that day.
- Ask everyone to share their proudest accomplishment over the past 30 days.
- Make a running list of your family's successes in the past week, even the smallest ones, and celebrate them (eg, dance, laugh, high five).

✔ **Activity for the week:** Make plans to incorporate as many of the following Activities for the Week that you reasonably can:

- Build a new memory with your child(ren) this week that you want to hold on to forever. Experience the moment fully.
- Map out your weekly meal plan (see the Weekly Meal Planner and recipe ideas in the Appendix).
- Map out your weekly fitness plan (see the Family Fit Tracker in the Appendix).
- Map out and post your family schedule.
- Self-monitor nutrition and physical activity. Consider using the Family Fit Tracker in the Appendix.

✔ **Closing family activity:** Close this week's meeting by taking a 5- to 10-minute savoring walk together.

Part 3
Post-plan

What causes a vegetable-averse teen to turn into a salad-loving adult? How do some busy families get into the habit of eating dinner together nearly every night, while it feels next to impossible for others? How is it that a person who started off disliking exercise later becomes a committed runner? The science is far from complete, but a growing body of research offers clues to piece together how some people make behavior changes that stick.

It seems to come down to a few factors: *the person, the goal, the program,* and *the environment.* Applying this understanding to your Family Fit Plan can help turn the changes you've made over the past 30 days into lasting lifestyle changes.

The "person" factors include beliefs about the 5 health areas (nutrition, exercise, sleep, screen time, and stress), expectations of what would occur with a change, the home environment, usual behaviors, and knowledge and skill in translating knowledge into daily behaviors. These are most of the things that you and your family have been working on over the past 4 weeks.

The "goal" factors include the seriousness and importance of your family's "why" that made you start the program in the first place whether that is a disease that is being treated or avoided or an outcome you hope to achieve, such as improved fitness, weight loss, better family relationships, or overall improved family happiness and health. You described your why as you planned for the Family Fit Plan.

The "program" factors refer to the difficulty, complexity, and extent of change required to meet your goals (or in our case, implement your Family Fit Plan). If you feel your plan has been easy to understand and follow, you are more likely to change. On the other hand, if it has been too complex and hard to follow, your changes likely won't stick.

The "environmental" factors include your family's environment at home, at school, work, or other community settings. The beliefs and culture around food, exercise, sleep, screen time, and how to cope with stress in these settings plays an important role in determining what changes you've made and those that you continue.

Taking these factors into account, the Post-plan: Making Changes That Stick chapter helps you transfer the positive momentum from the past month into continued change.

Post-plan: Making Changes That Stick

Congratulations on completing the Family Fit Plan! Hopefully, your family has adopted new routines that have boosted your family's health and fitness while having a little bit of fun at the same time. Now it's time to take a look back at the past month, see how your family has changed, and take steps to make those changes stick.

Family Fit Plan Check-in

At the end of week 4, you compared what was different in the 5 focus areas (nutrition, physical activity, sleep, screen time, and stress) between now and when you started the Family Fit Plan. It is now time to take a closer look at your progress and get a more complete sense of what has gone well over the past 30 days, including the goals that you have met and action plans you have completed, as well as goals still in progress and those you have abandoned. It also is a great time to reinforce systems and routines that will set your family on a continued path to better health and fitness. Reflect on your progress using the Mindful Moment: "Post–Family Fit Plan Check-in and Where to Go From Here" Box. What is different now? Did anyone's food preferences, likes, and dislikes change? Are your cooking skills better? Has your fitness improved? Have you developed a plan around screen time? Does anyone sleep better or manage stress in a more productive way?

Mindful Moment: Post-Family Fit Plan Check-in and Where to Go From Here

How did your family change over the last 30-days?

1. Look back at your Family Fit Plan SMART goals and action plans (see Chapter 3). How many of your action plans did you complete? How close are you to accomplishing your SMART goals?

2. Repeat the fitness assessment you completed at the onset of the Family Fit Plan. Use the Fitness Assessment Log in the Appendix to fill in your before and after measurements. How did your fitness change?

3. What was your biggest accomplishment?

4. What do you wish would have gone differently?

5. What would you like to focus on most now?

Now What?

Of course, this is not the end but, actually, a transition to the next phase of your journey. In this phase, you set new goals and action steps tailored to your vision for the future for optimal family health and fitness. Part of this transition is moving away from a mindset of precision and perfection to one that is sensitive to the ebb and flow of life. We acknowledge that as humans we make mistakes; we don't always follow through on our intentions, and sometimes, even despite our best efforts, unexpected challenges can get in our way, forcing us to take 1 or more steps back before we can leap forward again.

Create Your Family Rules to Live By

Now that you have made changes in the way that you and your family live and have invested time in figuring out what you want for your family, it may be a good time to create your Family Rules to Live By. These rules are principles that guide the way in which you would like to raise your family and teach your children how to be healthy and fit as well as be good citizens in your family and society. These principles may be different for every family. But defining them will help you create a strong set of traditions for your children and family, with memories and experiences that will stay with them through childhood and into adulthood when they raise their own families.

To help you get started, I will share with you what my family has adopted as our rules to live by.

1. We eat most meals together, at the table, with no distractions.
2. We model respect and good manners.
3. We follow our routines and schedules predictably but not rigidly.
4. We respect each other and each other's preferences, although we do not necessarily cater to them.
5. We strive for balance and moderation in most things, most of the time.
6. We use food as fuel, and not as a comfort or reward.
7. We embrace movement and physical activity as a gift to treasure, and not a punishment.
8. We strive to succeed and use setbacks and failures as opportunities to build our strength and resilience.
9. We practice mindfulness.
10. We celebrate success.

Your family does not have to adopt the same rules to be successful. These rules are just an example of the types of factors to take into account. The rules my family has adopted are based on research and advice from experts I trust, a lot of parents and families in my pediatrics practice, and trial and error.

Being Open to Change

Whether or not you've run into any lapses so far, the reality of making any behavioral change is that disruptors sometimes get in the way. Lapses are normal and expected. You can boost the chances that your family's healthier habits will stick (and prevent a full relapse, or return to your starting behavior—your life before the Family Fit Plan), by incorporating as many of the following 12 research-proven strategies into your plan as possible:

1. Check readiness.

Different family members may be in different stages of readiness to make the changes over the past month permanent. Recognizing this can help you to tailor your approach. For example, some studies show that adherence to change is poor when people are not really motivated to change, do not have family support, or have negative feelings about the change they are being asked to make. On the other hand, people most likely to stick with a change are already in the midst of making changes and had better nutrition and activity habits at the start. Think of family members who were most enthusiastic about this plan. They are likely to keep up the motivation. On the other hand, those family members who were most reluctant or uninterested in changing will be most likely to revert to the old ways or intentionally or unintentionally undermine the efforts of other family members.

2. Avoid lecturing.

Rather than lecturing or providing lots of information on why good nutrition and fitness habits are important, try a new approach. First, use open-ended questions to understand what a family member already knows. For example, ask your child, "What do you know about fruit?" Let your child answer, and then ask if it's OK if you share a little bit of information to build on what your child knows. Ask your child how this information might be useful in his or her life. For example, I took this approach with my own kids (ages 10 and 7) and asked them, "What do you know about fruit?" They said they know that fruits are nutritious and healthy, they contain seeds, and they are delicious (except for tomatoes, says the 10-year-old who is still training his taste buds to like them). I asked them if it would be OK if I tell them something else about fruits that they might not already know. They agreed, so I told them that fruits have lots of fiber. I shared with them that fiber helps us to feel full. Then I asked them why knowing all this about fruits matters. The 7-year-old answered, "So that I will know how good they are for me when I see them, and so I will eat more of them!" Her saying that helped her to strengthen her positive feelings toward fruits. If I had said it or lectured her why it's so important that she eats fruits, she would be more likely to resist them. By saying it herself, she may actually be more likely to eat them when they are available.

3. Be flexible.

Be flexible in your nutrition and fitness recommendations or action steps for the family. Take into account food and activity preferences and try to be accommodating without becoming a short-order cook. For example, when making dinners, choose 1 food that you know a more reluctant family member will like. When deciding on family physical activities, ask for ideas and suggestions. Discourage eating desserts every day, but at the same time, don't completely restrict not-so-healthy favorite foods. Rather, help kids learn how they can fit them into an overall healthy living plan.

4. Self-monitor.

Self-monitoring is one of the most important factors to improve adherence to nutrition and exercise recommendations. Keep in place systems that help family members keep tabs on their own nutrition and fitness ventures. This could be as simple as keeping a weekly meal planner where you map out family meals and snacks and a fitness tracker where everyone records their daily exercise. Tools to help you do this are included in the Appendix.

5. Keep setting SMART goals with associated action steps.

For the 30 days of the Family Fit Plan you set SMART goals. Now keep it going. You started with small, fairly easy-to-achieve behavior-oriented goals that focus on adding a new desired behavior, rather than taking away an old behavior. This helps create early successful experiences. For example, you may have had a SMART goal to eat a fruit or vegetable at each meal for the next week. The success from achieving a SMART goal sets the stage for continued success. Build SMART goals onto each other until the new behavior is a normal habit. Use fitness-related SMART goals to reach new achievements. For example, I set a personal SMART goal to be able to do 1 unassisted pull-up by the end of the year (something that has been very elusive for me!). My action step was to practice 10 band-assisted pull-ups every day. Without a SMART goal and associated action steps, I'm pretty sure I would never have achieved that feat! For many families, the way to make the changes stick and continue to grow is to repeat the Family Fit Plan. Your family can achieve new goals and new levels of fitness, happiness, and health each time you go through a 4-week cycle.

6. List the factors that make your changes easier and those that make them more difficult.

Going through this process helps to clearly identify strong supports for making the nutrition change as well as barriers to change. After you have considered the barriers, make a list of ways you might overcome them.

7. Prepare for lapses.

Lapses are a normal part of making any behavior change. No behavior change is ever perfect. If you expect lapses, they will be less likely to throw you off when they occur. Everyone knows of a person who tried a diet only to abandon the new behaviors after a slipup. The thinking goes something like this: "I've already screwed it up anyway; I might as well just eat whatever I want now." Or a family may have made healthful changes, only to go on vacation and abandon most of the healthful changes (as many people do on vacation). They return home committed to return to the healthful behaviors but are not confident they will be able to sustain them. These blips are normal and expected. Be aware of when they are happening, and have a plan for getting back on track so that they are just temporary slipups.

An important strategy to help do this is to identify high-risk situations that are likely to trigger lapses before the lapse actually occurs. For many families, common lapses include life events such as an injury that impedes physical activity, a vacation in which eating in restaurants and in excess are common, a job change that can disrupt individual and family routines, and summer breaks and school changes.

Once you've identified high-risk situations, take a few minutes to try to understand what makes them challenging. For example, ask yourself (or your family members) the following questions:

- What is the hardest part about continuing these nutrition changes?
- What is it that makes it so difficult to add in 30 minutes of physical activity most days?
- Why do I keep picking up my phone off the nightstand when I can't fall asleep at night, even though I know that it makes my sleep worse?
- Why is it so hard to get a healthy meal on the table each night?

After asking these questions, brainstorm potential solutions to the problem. Think about a time in the past when you had the same or similar difficulty and how you overcame it. What might make it easier to continue the changes you've started over the past 4 weeks? How might you address the 2 or 3 biggest problems that will get in your way?

Make a list of potential solutions. Consider the likely positive and negative outcomes from each of your potential solutions and then choose 1. You can do this in the form of a SMART goal solution with several action steps to implement the plan. For example, "I stopped exercising because I got too busy and just couldn't fit it into my day. When this happened in the past, I started walking around the field when my kids were at soccer practice. I had to be there anyway, so it didn't take any more time out of my day. I guess that I could try doing this again. The downside is I don't get to see them practice or socialize with the other parents. But the upside is that I get my exercise in without feeling stressed that I should be doing something else. For the next month, when my kids are at sports practice, instead of sitting on the sidelines, I will walk around the field for at least 30 minutes of each practice."

Then, implement your plan by either avoiding or coping with the potential or actual triggers, using your SMART plan to avoid a full relapse (ie, a return to your old habits). Evaluate your plan by assessing how well the solution helped to solve the problem. If it was not effective, start again by exploring other possible solutions.

8. Take advantage of every opportunity to improve cooking skills.

One study looked at how well fifth graders and their parents were able to stick to the dietary recommendations for milk, whole grains, fruits, and vegetables. The study found that 1 of the biggest barriers for the adults was lack of skills in meal prepping and preparing recipes. Hopefully, you were able to improve your cooking skills throughout the 30 days of the Family Fit Plan. Keep the momentum going by continuing to practice with the recipes and learn new tricks. A few excellent resources include ChopChop Family (https://www.chopchopfamily.org), US Department of Agriculture What's Cooking (https://whatscooking.fns.usda.gov), Food Network (https://www.foodnetwork.com), and Epicurious (https://www.epicurious.com).

9. Take advantage of every opportunity to increase the amount of movement in your day.

Increased levels of physical activity are easier to keep up when they occur as part of everyday life. Continue to park in the farthest spots in parking lots, take the stairs instead of the elevator, and prioritize active family adventures and together time.

10. Build in accountability.

Create an accountability plan that will help you stay on track. This might be keeping your Family Fit Plan in a visible place, committing to other family members or friends to work out together, or posting a weekly meal plan that your family members expect to stick with for the most part.

11. Build in social support.

Social support is a critical factor in sustaining any type of behavior change. In fact, it is so important, the first chapter of this book includes a heavy focus on growing and nurturing your social supports.

12. Model the change you want your family to make.

We've discussed this one a lot during the Family Fit Plan, but it's worth mentioning again. The best way to positively influence the rest of the family is to model the changes you'd like them to make. At the same time, be flexible with yourself and recognize that lapses occur for all of us. Models who already practice the goal behavior are very motivating for others, especially if the model is considered to be trustworthy, admirable, and respected. Also, the modeled behavior needs to be perceived as achievable. In addition to serving as a positive model for the rest of your family, also seek out models and mentors that help to inspire you and your family to continue on your journey.

Family Meeting: Making Changes That Stick

Now that you and your family have completed your 30-day Family Fit Plan, you will decide together this week what your next steps will be.

✔ Open the meeting by asking family members what area of health they feel that they improved the most over the course of the plan: nutrition, physical activity, sleep, screen time, or stress management? Why do they feel that way?

✔ **Activity:** Choose one of the following activities to do during your family meeting:
- Complete the Mindful Moment: "Post–Family Fit Plan Check-in and Where to Go From Here" Box.
- Make a list of your Family Rules to Live By.
- Ask everyone to share 1 thing that they changed over the past month that they are most proud of and would like to keep as a new habit.
- Go through the process for preparing for lapses.
- Create an accountability plan.

✔ **Activity for the week:** Make plans to incorporate as many of the following Activities for the Week that you reasonably can:
- Complete the Mindful Moment: "Post–Family Fit Plan Check-in and Where to Go From Here" fitness assessment and compare your results now with your results before you started the plan.
- Map out your weekly meal plan (see the Weekly Meal Planner and recipe ideas in the Appendix).
- Map out your weekly fitness plan (see the Family Fit Tracker in the Appendix).
- Map out and post your family schedule.
- Self-monitor nutrition and physical activity. Consider using the Family Fit Tracker in the Appendix.

✔ **Closing family activity:** High fives all around! End the family meeting by playing a "high fives" game in which each family member says something positive about a change another family member made over the past month and gives him or her a high five. For example, a teen might say, "Mom, you made and taught me how to make some really awesome and healthy dinners!" Follow that with a high five.

You are well on your way to continue your new beginning! Hopefully you feel armed with the knowledge, tools, and resources you need to transform your 30-day plan into continued lifestyle change. And most importantly, I hope you and your family enjoy the journey. Thank you for taking part in the Family Fit Plan.

Appendix

Recipes, Reinforcement Planners, and Workouts

---

*These recipes can help bring your Family Fit Plan to life. They were all created by pediatrician Mary Saph Tanaka, MD, MS, and first appeared in the book *"Eat Your Vegetables" and Other Mistakes Parents Make: Redefining How to Raise Healthy Eaters.*

135

Recipes

Breakfast

Choose Your Own Oatmeal

Ingredients:

2 cups uncooked oats

3 cups water (or milk for thicker consistency)

½ teaspoon salt

Crushed almonds and/or walnuts

SERVES
4

Directions:

1. Bring water or milk and salt to boil over medium heat. Add oats and stir. Lower heat and cook uncovered for 8 to 10 minutes or until most of the liquid is absorbed, stirring occasionally.

2. Keep it interesting with the following variations:

★ **"Banana Bread" Oatmeal:** Add 1 tablespoon of cinnamon and 1 tablespoon of brown sugar or honey to water or milk and bring to boil. Peel 2 ripe bananas into a bowl and mash with a fork. After you add the oats to the water or milk, add the bananas to the oatmeal and stir. Lower heat and cook uncovered for 8 to 10 minutes, stirring occasionally. Top with chopped toasted walnuts.

★ **Cinnamon Apple Oatmeal:** Dice 2 apples into ¼-inch pieces and place into a pot over medium heat. In a separate bowl, add 1 tablespoon of cinnamon and 2 tablespoons of brown sugar or honey to the water or milk, then pour mixture over the apples. Bring the mixture to a boil and then lower the heat. Add the oats and stir. Lower the heat and cook uncovered for 8 to 10 minutes, stirring occasionally.

★ **Strawberries and Cream Oatmeal:** Cook basic oatmeal as instructed in the "Choose Your Own Oatmeal." Add ½ cup of nonfat milk to the oatmeal and stir. Add ¼ cup of strawberry jam/preserves to the oatmeal and stir. Lower the heat, and cook uncovered for 3 to 4 minutes, stirring occasionally. Serve with a dollop of strawberry jam on top.

★ **Peanut Butter and Jelly Oatmeal:** Cook basic oatmeal as instructed in the "Choose Your Own Oatmeal." When serving the oatmeal, place 1 tablespoon of jelly and 1 tablespoon of peanut butter on top of the oatmeal.

TIP: Make a large batch of oatmeal and transfer serving-size amounts to a muffin tin greased with nonstick cooking spray. Freeze the tray and, once frozen, transfer the servings to an airtight freezer bag. Then, when you are ready to eat, simply empty the oatmeal from the freezer bag to a pan greased with nonstick spray and warm up on the stove or microwave the oatmeal in a bowl on high for 1 to 2 minutes. Add your favorite toppings, and you're good to go!

Green Chia Smoothie

Ingredients:

1 banana

2 cups baby spinach (washed and dried)

1 cup frozen peaches

1 cup frozen pineapples

2 teaspoons chia seeds

1 cup unsweetened almond milk

SERVES
4

Directions:

Blend all ingredients well until smooth. Divide into 4 glasses and serve.

Yogurt Parfait

Ingredients:

2 cups plain nonfat yogurt

1 cup fruit mixture (include your favorites such as strawberries, blueberries, raspberries, blackberries, chopped banana, etc)

1 cup Coconutty Blueberry Granola

SERVES
4

Directions:

To prepare parfaits, place ¼ cup of yogurt at the bottom of a sundae glass. Place 1 tablespoon of the fruit mixture over the yogurt. Place another ¼ cup of yogurt on top, followed by 1 more tablespoon of the fruit mixture. Sprinkle ¼ cup of the granola on top.

Goin' Nuts and Bananas! (Peanut Butter Banana Pancakes)

SERVES
4

Ingredients:

1 cup whole wheat flour

1 cup rolled oats

1 teaspoon baking soda

1 teaspoon baking powder

¼ cup brown sugar

3 ripe bananas, mashed

½ cup buttermilk or plain yogurt

¼ cup peanut butter

2 eggs

2 tablespoons butter, melted

1 tablespoon cinnamon

1 teaspoon salt

1 tablespoon vanilla extract

Toppings

Banana chips

Walnuts

Peanut butter

Directions:

1. **To prepare the wet ingredients:** Crack the eggs into a medium mixing bowl and beat lightly. Add the melted butter and peanut butter and then whisk until well incorporated. Mix in the brown sugar and stir. Add the buttermilk/yogurt and vanilla to the egg mixture and stir. Add the mashed bananas and stir until incorporated.

2. **To prepare dry ingredients:** Blend rolled oats in a blender until fine and then pour into a separate bowl. Add the whole wheat flour, baking soda, baking powder, salt, and cinnamon to the bowl and stir. Pour half of the dry ingredients into the wet ingredients and fold gently. Add the remaining dry ingredients and gently fold until just incorporated.

3. Spray a shallow pan with nonstick cooking spray and place over low-medium heat. Pour approximately ¼ cup of the batter into the pan. Cook for 3 to 4 minutes or until the top of the pancake has bubbles. Flip the pancake and cook for another 3 to 4 minutes. Remove from heat. Add crushed banana chips and walnuts and a dollop of peanut butter on top of the pancakes and serve.

Coconutty Blueberry Granola

Ingredients:

3 cups rolled oats

1 cup pecans, chopped

1 cup cashews, chopped

1½ cups dried blueberries

1½ cups shredded coconut

1 teaspoon salt

1 tablespoon ground cinnamon

1 tablespoon vanilla extract

½ cup brown sugar

3 tablespoons butter, melted

3 tablespoons brown rice syrup or honey

SERVES
4

Directions:

Preheat the oven to 325°F. Mix all ingredients together in a large mixing bowl and pour evenly on to an ungreased baking sheet. Bake for 20 minutes and then remove from the oven and stir. Place back into the oven and cook for another 15 minutes. Remove the pan from the oven and stir. Let cool to room temperature. Serve with milk or yogurt.

Whole-Grain Waffle Apple Peanut Butter Sandwiches

Ingredients:

4 frozen whole-grain waffles, defrosted

8 tablespoons peanut butter

2 apples

SERVES
4

Directions:

Toast the waffles until golden brown. Cut each apple in half, remove the core, and cut the apples into thin slices. Evenly spread 2 tablespoons of peanut butter on each waffle. Add sliced apples to two of the waffles and cover with the remaining two waffles. Cut each "waffle sandwich" in half.

Frittata Muffins

SERVES 4

Ingredients:

4 eggs

1 cup assorted vegetables, chopped into small pieces

¼ cup nonfat milk

2 teaspoons salt

2 teaspoons black pepper

Directions:

1. Preheat the oven to 375°F. Crack the eggs into a medium-sized bowl and beat lightly. Add the milk into the eggs and stir. Add the vegetables into the bowl and stir gently. Sprinkle in the salt and pepper.

2. Spray a muffin tin with nonstick cooking spray, and line it with cupcake liners. Pour the egg mixture into each muffin compartment, until approximately ¾ full. Bake for about 15 minutes. Makes approximately 10 to 12 muffins.

TIPS: For breakfast: Cut 1 muffin into slices and put the slices between 2 pieces of whole wheat toast for a healthy breakfast sandwich.

For lunch: Serve a frittata with a green salad for a balanced lunch.

Lunch

Creamy Roasted Red Pepper Tomato Soup (With Spinach Grilled Cheese)

SERVES 4

Ingredients:

2 15-ounce cans chopped tomatoes

3 red bell peppers

1 medium yellow onion, diced

2 garlic cloves, chopped

3 tablespoons tomato paste

1 medium Yukon Gold potato

3 cups water

Directions:

1. Wash and dry all the vegetables. To prepare the roasted red peppers, preheat the oven to 400°F. Place the washed red peppers on a baking sheet and bake for approximately 30 minutes. Once the skin is blistered or charred, remove the peppers from the oven and place them in a bowl. Cover with plastic wrap and let cool for 15 minutes.

2. While the peppers are roasting and cooling, prepare the other soup ingredients. Dice the medium onion and garlic into small pieces and set aside. Wash the potato and scrub the skin. Cut the potato into ½-inch chunks. Heat 2 tablespoons of olive oil in a large pot over medium heat. Place the onions and garlic into the pot and stir. Once the onions and garlic are slightly browned, add the potatoes, chopped tomatoes, and tomato paste and stir. Remove the peppers from the bowl, peel the charred skin, remove the seeds, and place the peppers into the pot. Add the water and let simmer for 40 minutes, stirring occasionally. Remove the pot from the heat and let cool for 15 minutes. In batches, transfer the soup to a blender and blend until smooth. Serve with spinach grilled cheese.

Ingredients:

8 pieces whole-grain bread

2 cups shredded cheddar cheese

2 cups baby spinach

Olive oil

Directions:

Preheat the oven to 375°F. Place the bread on a baking sheet and brush both sides of each slice lightly with olive oil. Place ¼ cup of cheddar cheese on 4 slices of the bread. Next, place ½ cup of baby spinach on top of the cheese, and then sprinkle another ¼ cup of the cheese on top of the spinach. Place the remaining slices of bread on top of the spinach and cheese to make 4 sandwiches. Bake for 10 minutes. Remove the baking sheet from the oven and, using a spatula, press down on each sandwich. Flip each sandwich onto the other side and place the baking sheet back into the oven for 10 minutes. Remove the baking sheet from the oven and slice each sandwich in half diagonally.

Creamy Cauliflower Soup

Ingredients:

1 head cauliflower, cut into small florets

1 medium white onion, diced

1 medium potato, cut into ¼-inch cubes

2 cloves garlic, chopped

1 teaspoon ground cumin

½ teaspoon salt

¼ teaspoon pepper

SERVES **4**

Directions:

1. Heat a large pot over medium heat. Place 2 tablespoons of olive oil into the pot and add the onion pieces. Cook the onion pieces for 5 minutes and add the cauliflower, potato, and garlic. Sprinkle in the cumin, salt, and pepper. Add water to the pot to cover the vegetables by approximately ½ inch. Bring the water to a boil and then turn the heat to low and let simmer for 40 minutes.

2. Turn off the stove, remove the pot from the heat, and let it cool approximately 10 minutes. Blend the soup in batches (taking care while removing the lid of the blender because of hot steam). Ladle the soup into bowls and serve.

TIP: Don't have cauliflower? Substitute it with broccoli for a creamy broccoli soup.

Tuna Salad Lettuce Wraps

Ingredients:

2 8-ounce cans tuna, drained

1 15-ounce can white cannellini
    beans, drained

2 celery ribs, diced

½ medium red onion, diced

¼ cup sun-dried tomatoes, julienned

¼ cup black olives, sliced in half

¼ cup Italian parsley, chopped

2 tablespoons olive oil

Juice of ½ lemon

1 teaspoon salt and pepper

½ head red leaf lettuce, washed and dried

SERVES **4**

Directions:

Mix all ingredients, except lettuce, together in a bowl and stir. Serve the mixture on top of lettuce leaves.

Rainbow Pinwheels

Ingredients:

2 whole wheat tortillas

1 cup baby spinach, washed and dried

6 slices of deli-sliced turkey breast

½ cup grated carrots

1 red bell pepper, seeded and julienned

½ cup shredded cheddar cheese

SERVES
2-4

Directions:

Place 1 tortilla in a pan over low heat. Sprinkle ¼ cup of cheddar cheese over the tortilla. Remove the tortilla from the heat once the cheese has melted and turn off the stove. Place ½ cup of spinach over the cheese in 1 layer and then cover the spinach with 3 slices of turkey breast. Next, place ½ of the carrots and bell pepper in a single layer on ½ of the tortilla. Starting at the end covered with the cheese, spinach, turkey, and vegetables, roll the tortilla into a burrito. Slice into 1-inch rounds. Repeat this procedure with the second tortilla.

Mean Green Pita Pockets

Ingredients:

2 loaves whole wheat pita bread

1 cup cheddar cheese

1 cup broccoli florets

1 chicken breast (see Simple Baked Chicken Breast in the Dinner section of this Appendix)

1 carrot, peeled and grated

SERVES
2-4

Directions:

1. Preheat the oven to 375°F. Shred the chicken breast into small pieces using a fork (or your hands if the chicken is cool to the touch). Place the shredded chicken into a bowl. Chop broccoli florets into small pieces and add them to the bowl. Stir the grated carrot into the bowl and mix well.

2. Split 1 pita bread loaf into 2 pieces. Sprinkle ¼ cup of cheddar cheese on one side of the pita bread. Place approximately ½ cup of the chicken and vegetable mixture on top of the cheese. Sprinkle with another ¼ cup of cheddar cheese. Place the remaining pita half on top and gently press to flatten the filling inside. Repeat with the second pita bread loaf. Reserve the remaining filling in the refrigerator.

3. Place the prepared pita bread loaves on an ungreased baking sheet and bake for 15 minutes. Remove the baking sheet from the oven, cut each pita sandwich in half, and serve.

Balsamic Roasted Vegetables (and Caramelized Onion Couscous Salad)

Balsamic Roasted Vegetables

½ head cauliflower, cut into small florets

2 cups brussels sprouts, halved

2 cups butternut squash, cut into ½-inch cubes

4 tablespoons olive oil

4 tablespoons balsamic vinegar

½ teaspoon salt

¼ teaspoon pepper

Caramelized Onion Couscous Salad

1 medium onion

1 cup dried couscous

1½ cups water

Directions:

To prepare the roasted vegetables, preheat the oven and an ungreased baking sheet to 375°F. Place the cauliflower, brussels sprouts, and butternut squash into a bowl. Mix in the olive oil, balsamic vinegar, and salt and pepper until the vegetables are coated. Pour the vegetables onto the baking sheet in a single layer. Bake for approximately 30 minutes, until the vegetables are tender and browned.

TIP: While root vegetables such as potatoes, parsnips, carrots, and squash are the most commonly roasted vegetables, almost any vegetable tastes delicious roasted. Just experiment and see which ones your family enjoys most.

To prepare the onion couscous salad, cut the onion in half, and then cut into thin slices. On the stovetop, heat a pot over medium heat. Place 2 tablespoons of olive oil into the pot and add the onion slices. Cook the onion for approximately 10 minutes, stirring occasionally, until soft and browned. Add the water to the pot with onions, taking care while pouring the water, as it might spatter. Bring the water to a boil and then add the couscous to the pot. Immediately cover the pot with the lid and turn off the heat. Move to a cool spot and let sit for 7 minutes. Then remove the lid and fluff the couscous with a fork.

To serve, place 1 cup of couscous on a plate and cover it with approximately 1 cup of the vegetable mixture.

Optional: Sprinkle 1 tablespoon of goat cheese on top of the vegetables and serve.

Cold Sesame Whole Wheat Noodle and Kale Salad

SERVES
4

Ingredients:

½ package whole wheat spaghetti

1 red bell pepper, seeded and julienned

1 bunch kale, destemmed and leaves
   cut into ½-inch ribbons

½ cup chopped cilantro

¼ cup soy sauce

Juice of 1 orange

2 tablespoons sesame seeds

3 tablespoons olive oil

Directions:

Bring a large pot of water to a boil. Add the spaghetti to the water and cook according to instructions on the package. At approximately 5 minutes prior to the end of the pasta's cooking time, add the kale to the water and cook for 5 minutes. Drain the mixture into a colander and put it into a large mixing bowl. Add the bell pepper julienned strips to the kale/pasta mixture. Pour the soy sauce, orange juice, sesame seeds, and olive oil into the bowl and mix until well coated. Add chopped cilantro and serve.

Dinner

Mix-and-Match Dinners by Food Group

protein

Simple Baked Chicken Breast

Ingredients:

4 boneless, skinless chicken breasts
1 tablespoon olive oil

1 teaspoon salt
½ teaspoon pepper

SERVES
4

Directions:

Preheat the oven to 350°F. Place the chicken breasts on a baking sheet, and drizzle them with olive oil, salt, and pepper. Bake for 30 to 45 minutes or until thoroughly cooked.

TIP: Make extra chicken and use in sandwiches, tacos, and wraps for the rest of the week.

Perfect Steamed Fish

Ingredients:

4 ounces fish fillet
½ teaspoon salt
¼ teaspoon pepper

2 tablespoons water, lemon juice, orange juice, or soy sauce

SERVES
4

Directions:

1. Preheat the oven to 350°F. Tear a piece of foil approximately 3 times the size of the fish fillet. Place the 4-ounce fillet in the center of the foil. Sprinkle fish with salt and pepper. Bring up all sides of the foil perpendicular to the fish (as if creating 4 walls). Place 2 tablespoons of liquid (eg, water, lemon juice, orange juice, or soy sauce) on top of the fish. Bring 2 opposite sides of the foil together in the middle and roll down until it meets the fish. Roll the remaining sides of the foil into the center, which creates a package where the fish is completely enclosed.

2. Place on an ungreased baking sheet and bake for 20 to 25 minutes.

TIP: Add julienned vegetables on top of the fish before cooking for an easy and quick meal.

Flavorful Tofu

Ingredients:

1 package extra-firm tofu

1 cup marinade (of your choosing)

2 tablespoons olive oil

SERVES
4

Directions:

Using the extra-firm variety of tofu, cut the tofu into ½-inch slabs. Marinate the tofu in any spice mixture or sauce overnight so the tofu absorbs the flavor. The next day, place 2 tablespoons of olive oil in a pan over medium heat, and pan fry the tofu for 6 to 7 minutes on each side.

TIP: Try marinating with barbecue sauce for a healthier alternative in sandwiches.

vegetables

Easy Cooked Vegetables

Ingredients:

1 head cauliflower, trimmed and cut into small florets

1 medium-sized potato, washed and cut into ½-inch cubes

¼ cup low-fat plain yogurt

1 teaspoon salt

½ teaspoon pepper

Directions:

Place cauliflower and potatoes into a pot. Add water until the vegetables are completely covered. Bring the water to a boil and then reduce to medium heat and cook for 20 to 30 minutes. Once the vegetables are tender, remove them from the heat and mash them with a potato masher or fork. Add ¼ cup of yogurt, salt, and pepper.

Crispy Green Bean "Fries"

Ingredients:

1 pound green beans

2 tablespoons olive oil

1 teaspoon salt

½ teaspoon pepper

Directions:

Preheat the oven to 425°F. Place the green beans on an ungreased baking sheet in a single layer and sprinkle olive oil over the green beans. Sprinkle salt and pepper. Bake for 20 minutes, until crispy.

Baked Sweet Potato Fries

Ingredients:

3 medium-sized sweet potatoes

2 tablespoons olive oil

SERVES
3

Directions:

Preheat the oven to 450°F. Wash the sweet potatoes well. Cut into ⅛-inch round slices and put them into a bowl. Drizzle 2 tablespoons of olive oil on top of the potatoes and mix well until the potatoes are coated. Place the potatoes on an ungreased baking sheet in a single layer and bake for approximately 25 minutes or until crispy and brown.

TIPS: Enjoy pumpkin pie? Try adding cinnamon and nutmeg to the potatoes.

Enjoy southwestern flavors? Try adding cumin and garlic to the potatoes.

Roasted Garlicky and Cheesy Broccoli

Ingredients:

1 head broccoli, trimmed and cut into florets

3 cloves garlic, cut into thin slices

¼ cup shredded Parmesan cheese

Olive oil

Salt and pepper

Directions:

Preheat the oven to 375°F. Toss the broccoli florets with 3 tablespoons of olive oil, garlic, salt, and pepper. Spread broccoli in an even layer on a baking sheet. Bake for 20 minutes. Remove from oven and sprinkle cheese on the broccoli before serving.

Cucumber and Carrot Sesame Salad

Ingredients:

2 medium-sized carrots

1 large cucumber

1 to 2 stalks green onions, chopped

1 tablespoon sesame seeds

2 tablespoons vinegar or juice of 1 lime

1 teaspoon salt

½ teaspoon pepper

Directions:

Peel carrots and slice them in half lengthwise. Lay the carrots flat and cut into thin slices across. Put the carrots into a large bowl. Next, cut the cucumber in half lengthwise. Using a spoon, scrape out the seeds and then lay the cucumber flat and cut it into thin slices across. Place the cucumber into the bowl with the carrots and add green onions and sesame seeds. Mix in the vinegar or lime juice and stir. Add salt and pepper.

Corn and Black Bean Salad

Ingredients:

2 cups cooked brown rice

1 package frozen corn, defrosted

1 15-ounce can black beans, drained

1 medium cucumber

1 red bell pepper

½ cup cilantro (or green onions)

Juice of 1 lime

Salt and pepper

Directions:

Slice the cucumber in half lengthwise and scoop out the seeds with a spoon. Lay the cucumber flat and cut it across into thin slices. Cut the red bell pepper in half and remove the seeds. Dice the red pepper into small pieces. Place the cucumber and red bell pepper in a mixing bowl. Add the brown rice, corn, beans, cilantro and lime juice. Add salt and pepper as needed. Mix well.

carbohydrates

Basic Quinoa

Ingredients:

1 cup dry quinoa

2 cups water

Directions:

In a medium-sized pot, bring the water to a boil. Add the quinoa, cover the pot, and lower the heat to low-medium. Cook for 20 minutes.

Basic Whole Wheat Couscous

Ingredients:

1 cup dry couscous

1½ cups water

Directions:

In a medium-sized pot, bring the water to a boil. Add couscous, cover the pot, and turn off the heat. Let the couscous stand for 10 minutes and then fluff the couscous with a fork.

Basic Barley

Ingredients:

1 cup barley

2 cups water

Directions:

In a medium-sized pot, bring the water to a boil. Add the barley, cover the pot, and lower the heat to low-medium. Cook for 30 minutes. Drain the excess water from the barley.

TIPS:

★ Add any of these grains to a salad for a heartier meal.

★ Substitute chicken or vegetable broth for a tastier grain!

Dinner

Dinners With Food Groups Combined

Baked Honey Mustard Chicken Fingers With Apples and Carrots

Ingredients:

2 cups crispy brown rice cereal

3 boneless, skinless chicken breasts

2 teaspoons dried parsley or oregano

¼ cup Dijon mustard

3 tablespoons honey

Salt and pepper

Olive oil

**SERVES
4**

Directions:

1. Preheat the oven to 400°F. Cut the chicken breasts lengthwise into ¼-inch strips. Sprinkle the chicken strips with salt, pepper, and the dried parsley or oregano. Mix the mustard and honey together in a bowl, and pour the mixture into a large resealable plastic bag. Place the chicken strips in the bag and seal. Gently shake the bag to lightly coat the chicken strips on both sides with the mustard/honey mixture.

2. Place the cereal into another large resealable plastic bag. Gently crush the cereal into smaller bits (but not into a flour-like consistency). Transfer 4 to 5 chicken strips at a time from the mustard/honey mixture into the bag with the cereal. Coat the chicken with cereal and then place the chicken pieces approximately 2 inches apart on a baking sheet that has been sprayed with nonstick cooking spray. Drizzle 2 tablespoons of olive oil over the chicken and bake for approximately 20 to 25 minutes (depending on the thickness of the chicken pieces). Serve with apple slices and raw carrot sticks.

Chicken Tacos With Pico de Gallo and Elote (Mexican Corn on the Cob)

SERVES
4

Chicken Tacos

8 corn tortillas

2 large boneless, skinless chicken breasts

Mexican Spice Marinade

2 tablespoons olive oil

1 teaspoon ground cumin

1 teaspoon dried onion

1 teaspoon ground oregano

½ cup fresh cilantro

Pico de Gallo

¼ medium onion, finely chopped

4 tomatoes, chopped

1 large cucumber, seeded and chopped

½ cup fresh cilantro, chopped

Juice of 1 lime

1 teaspoon salt

½ teaspoon pepper

Elote

4 ears of fresh corn, husks removed

3 tablespoons Greek yogurt

1 tablespoon mayonnaise

¼ cup grated Parmesan cheese

1 teaspoon cayenne pepper (optional)

1 lime, quartered

Directions:

1. *To prepare the chicken:* Mix together the olive oil, dried onion, and spices to make the Mexican Spice Marinade, and marinate the chicken breasts for at least 1 hour. Preheat the oven to 350°F. Place the chicken breasts on an ungreased baking sheet and bake for 30 to 45 minutes.

2. *To prepare the pico de gallo:* Mix the chopped tomatoes, onion, cucumber, and cilantro in a bowl. Add the juice of 1 lime. Sprinkle with salt and pepper.

3. *To prepare the elote:* Bring a large pot of water to boil. Place the corn into the boiling water and cook for approximately 5 minutes. Remove the corn from the water. Next, place an ungreased pan over medium heat. Once the pan is hot, put the corn in the pan and cook for 3 to 4 minutes on each side or until the kernels are slightly charred. In a small bowl, mix together the Greek yogurt, mayonnaise, and cayenne pepper (if using). Remove the corn from the pan and let it cool slightly. Spread 1 tablespoon of the yogurt mixture on each ear of corn and then sprinkle with 1 tablespoon of grated Parmesan. Serve with lime wedges.

4. *To make the tacos:* Assemble the tacos by heating the corn tortillas in a pan or in the oven. Chop the chicken breasts into ¼-inch cubes. Place a small amount of chicken in the middle of a tortilla and top with pico de gallo. Serve tacos with elote on the side.

Moroccan Chicken With Raisin Couscous

**SERVES
4**

Moroccan Chicken

6 bone-in chicken thighs, with skin

1 medium onion, chopped

2 garlic cloves, finely chopped

1 lemon, cut into ¼-inch slices

½ cup green olives, pitted and halved

1 teaspoon ground cardamom

2 teaspoons cinnamon

2 teaspoons ground coriander

2 cups chicken or vegetable broth

1 teaspoon salt

½ teaspoon pepper

3 tablespoons olive oil

Raisin Couscous

1½ cups dry couscous

¾ cup water

½ cup raisins

½ cup fresh parsley, chopped

Directions:

1. *To prepare the chicken:* Heat a wide-bottomed pot over medium heat. Carefully add olive oil to the heated pot. Sprinkle the chicken with salt and pepper. Place the chicken skin-side down in the pot and cook for 6 minutes. Flip the chicken over and cook for another 5 minutes. Remove the chicken from the pot and set aside.

2. Place the onions, garlic, and spices in the pot and cook for approximately 5 minutes, stirring occasionally. Add the lemon slices and cook for another 2 to 3 minutes. Return the chicken to the pot in an even layer. Add the olives and the broth to the pot. Bring the mixture to a gentle boil, then turn the heat to low and let simmer for 25 minutes.

3. *To prepare the couscous:* Bring the water to a boil in a pot with a fitted lid. Once the water is boiling, add dry couscous and raisins to the pot, cover, and turn off the heat. Let the couscous sit for approximately 10 minutes and then remove the lid and fluff the couscous with a fork.

4. Place the chicken over the raisin couscous and top it with the chopped parsley.

Pineapple Teriyaki Chicken With Rice and Broccoli

SERVES
4

Ingredients:

8 chicken drumsticks or thighs

1 15-ounce can diced pineapples

1½ cups soy sauce

¼ cup honey

2 cloves garlic, chopped (or 1 tablespoon garlic powder)

1 tablespoon fresh ginger root, grated

Olive oil

Directions:

1. In a large bowl, mix 1 cup of the soy sauce, ginger, and garlic. Remove the pineapple pieces from the can, and pour the pineapple juice into the bowl with the soy sauce. Reserve the pineapple pieces in a separate container and refrigerate. Add the chicken to the bowl with the pineapple juice and soy sauce. Wrap the bowl with plastic wrap and let it sit in the refrigerator 1 to 2 hours or overnight.

2. *To prepare the chicken*: Preheat the oven to 400°F. Remove the chicken from the bowl and place it on a baking sheet that has been lined with foil. Drizzle the chicken with 2 tablespoons of olive oil. Bake for 35 to 40 minutes.

3. *To prepare the sauce*: Bring ½ cup of soy sauce and ¼ cup of honey to a boil over medium heat. Lower heat and simmer for 15 minutes. Add the reserved pineapple pieces to the cooked sauce.

4. Once the chicken is cooked, remove it from the oven and pour the soy sauce/honey/pineapple sauce over the cooked chicken. Serve with cooked brown rice and steamed broccoli.

Rosemary Apricot Pork Sliders With Apple Cabbage Slaw

Rosemary Apricot Pork Sliders

1 pork tenderloin, cut into ½-inch
   round slices

8 mini burger buns or dinner rolls

¼ cup apricot preserves

2 teaspoons Dijon mustard

2 tablespoons fresh rosemary, chopped

1 teaspoon salt

½ teaspoon pepper

SERVES
4

Apple Cabbage Slaw

1 apple (any variety)

½ head green or red cabbage

2 carrots, peeled and grated

2 stalks green onions

½ cup plain Greek yogurt

1 tablespoon mayonnaise

1 teaspoon salt

½ teaspoon pepper

Directions:

1. To prepare the sliders: Place the pork tenderloin slices in a medium bowl with the rosemary, mustard, and 2 tablespoons of the apricot preserves. Mix gently until the pork is covered by the mixture. Sprinkle salt and pepper over pork. Marinate the pork in the refrigerator for 15 to 20 minutes.

2. In a small bowl, mix the remaining apricot preserves with 1 tablespoon of water. Remove the pork from the refrigerator. Heat a pan over medium heat and add 2 tablespoons of olive oil. Once the oil is heated, place the pork slices in the pan approximately 2 inches apart. Let the pork slices cook for 7 minutes and flip them over. Brush the top of each slice with the remaining apricot preserves. Cook the pork slices for another 7 minutes and then remove them from the heat.

3. *To prepare the slaw:* Wash the cabbage and discard the outer leaves. Chop the cabbage into thin slices and place them in a mixing bowl, followed by the grated carrots. Wash and quarter the apple, and then cut out the core. Slice each quarter into thin slices and then into julienne strips, and place them in the bowl. Wash and cut off the ends of the green onions, then make thin slices from the entire length of the onion and add them to the bowl. Add the yogurt and mayonnaise and mix. Add salt and pepper to the slaw and mix well.

4. Assemble the sliders by placing the slaw on one side of each bun, and then top with the pork and the remaining half of the bun. Serve with apple cabbage slaw on the side.

Curry Salmon Tomato Kabobs and Vegetable Biryani

Curry Salmon Tomato Kabobs

1-pound salmon fillets, cut into
  1-inch cubes

1 cup plain nonfat yogurt

2 tablespoons curry powder

1-pint cherry tomatoes

Wooden skewers

SERVES
4

Vegetable Biryani

2 cups brown rice, cooked

2 cups chopped vegetables
  (zucchini, broccoli,
  cauliflower)

1 medium onion, chopped

1 teaspoon ground cumin

1 teaspoon ground cinnamon

1 teaspoon ground cardamom

2 garlic cloves, finely chopped

½ inch fresh ginger, grated (or 1 teaspoon of
  ginger powder)

1 teaspoon chili powder (optional)

½ cup fresh cilantro, chopped

2 tablespoons olive oil

Directions:

1. *To prepare the salmon:* Mix the salmon cubes with yogurt and curry powder in a mixing bowl. Refrigerate the salmon for 30 minutes.

2. Place approximately 4 to 5 pieces of salmon on each skewer, alternating with the cherry tomatoes. Preheat the oven to 375°F. Place the skewers on a greased baking sheet, approximately 2 inches apart. Bake for 20 to 25 minutes, until the salmon is well done.

3. *To prepare the biryani:* Wash and dry all of the vegetables. Put olive oil in a pan over medium heat. Sauté the onions and spices in the pan for 2 minutes. Add chopped vegetables and cook for 3 to 4 minutes. Add rice and stir until well combined. Remove from heat.

4. Place skewers over the rice, sprinkle with chopped cilantro, and serve. If serving younger children, remove the salmon and tomatoes from the skewer before serving.

Grilled Salmon Tacos With Mango Black Bean Salsa

SERVES
4

Salmon Tacos

2 6-ounce salmon fillets

8 corn tortillas

1 lime, cut into wedges

2 tablespoons olive oil

Mexican Spice Marinade

2 tablespoons olive oil

1 teaspoon ground cumin

1 teaspoon dried onion

1 teaspoon ground oregano

½ cup fresh cilantro

Mango Black Bean Salsa

2 small mangos or 1½ cups of defrosted frozen mangos

1 15-ounce can of black beans, drained

¼ medium onion (any color), finely diced

1 red bell pepper, finely diced

½ cup of fresh cilantro, chopped

Juice of 1 lime

Directions:

1. *To prepare the salsa:* If using fresh mangos, peel the skin and slice the fruit off on either side of the seed. Cut the mangos into small pieces, approximately the same size as the peppers and onions. Mix all the ingredients together in a bowl and set aside.

2. *To prepare the fish:* Prepare the marinade by mixing all of the spices in a large bowl and adding 2 tablespoons of olive oil. Cut the fish into ½-inch cubes and add to the marinade. Refrigerate the marinating fish for 1 hour. When ready to cook, put 2 tablespoons of olive oil in a pan over medium heat and add the fish. Cook for 10 to 12 minutes, stirring occasionally, until the fish has cooked through. Assemble the tacos by heating the corn tortillas in an ungreased pan or in the oven. Put a small amount of the fish on each tortilla and serve with the mango black bean salsa.

Mahi-mahi Pitas With Feta, Cucumber, and Tomato Salad

Mahi-mahi Pitas

2 6-ounce mahi-mahi fillets

4 loaves whole wheat pita bread

SERVES
4

Middle Eastern Spice Marinade

¼ cup plain nonfat yogurt

1 teaspoon ground dried garlic
   (or 1 tablespoon fresh garlic)

1 teaspoon dried onion

¼ cup fresh mint

1 teaspoon ground cumin

Pinch of saffron

2 tablespoons olive oil

Feta, Cucumber, and Tomato Salad

1 English cucumber, seeded and
   chopped into ⅛-inch cubes

3 Roma or vine-ripened tomatoes,
   seeded and chopped into
   ⅛-inch cubes

¼ cup crumbled feta cheese

½ red onion, chopped

½ cup black olives, seeded and halved

2 tablespoons olive oil

Directions:

1. *To prepare the fish:* Mix the spice marinade ingredients together in a mixing bowl. Cut the mahi-mahi fillets into ½-inch cubes and place in the marinade. Refrigerate for 1 hour.

2. *To prepare the salad:* Put all the ingredients except the oil in a mixing bowl and mix well. Drizzle with the olive oil and set aside.

3. When the fish is ready to cook, put 2 tablespoons of olive oil in a pan over medium heat. Place the fish in the pan and cook for 10 to 12 minutes or until the fish is cooked through. Divide the fish mixture into 4 servings and place on top of warm pita bread.

4. Top the fish and pita bread with the salad mixture.

Chicken Chili Baked Potatoes

Ingredients:

4 baking potatoes, washed

1 medium onion, chopped

2 celery ribs, chopped

2 carrots, peeled and chopped

1 green bell pepper, diced

2 cups broccoli, cut into small florets

2 medium zucchinis, cut into
    ¼-inch slices

4 links of chicken andouille sausage,
    chopped into ¼-inch slices

1 15-ounce can kidney beans, drained

2 15-ounce cans chopped tomatoes

2 cups water

1 small jar salsa

SERVES 4

Directions:

1. Scrub the outside of the potato well. Poke the potato with a fork in a few places.

2. *To prepare in a microwave:* Place potatoes in the microwave on a microwave-safe plate and cook on high for 10-12 minutes, flip the potatoes to the other side, and then cook for an additional 10-12 minutes (or until a fork can easily pierce the potato).

3. *To prepare in an oven:* Preheat the oven to 400°F. Place the potatoes in a baking pan and bake for 45 minutes or until a fork can easily pierce the potato.

4. *To prepare the chili:* Put 2 tablespoons of olive oil in a large pot over medium heat. Place the onions into the oil and cook for approximately 5 minutes. Add celery, carrots, and bell pepper and cook until the vegetables have softened. Next, add the chicken sausage and cook for 5 minutes. Add in half of the broccoli and zucchini, kidney beans, tomatoes, and water. Bring the mixture to a boil, then turn the heat down to low, and let the chili simmer for approximately 20 minutes.

5. *To prepare the toppings:* Bring a pot of water to a boil over medium-high heat. Add the cut-up broccoli and zucchini and cook for 1 minute. Drain the water and place the vegetables in a bowl.

6. Remove the potatoes from the oven. Cut the potatoes in half. Serve them covered with the broccoli/zucchini topping, chili, cheese, and salsa.

TIP: Like sour cream on your baked potato? Try nonfat or low-fat plain yogurt instead.

Spaghetti and (Spinach) Meatballs

Ingredients:

1-pound ground beef, chicken, or turkey

8 ounces frozen spinach, defrosted

2 carrots, peeled and grated

1 zucchini, grated

½ cup rolled oats

1 15-ounce can tomato sauce

1 16-ounce package whole wheat spaghetti

2 tablespoons olive oil

1 teaspoon salt

2 teaspoons pepper

SERVES
6

Directions:

1. *To make the pasta:* Cook the pasta according to the instructions on the package.

2. *To make the meatballs:* Place the oats into a blender and blend until roughly chopped. Squeeze out all of the water from the defrosted spinach using your hands or a kitchen towel. Place the meat, spinach, and oatmeal in a large mixing bowl, and stir the contents to mix well. Add salt and pepper. Roll 1 spoonful of the mixture into a meatball and set aside. Continue making meatballs from the rest of the meat/vegetable mixture.

3. Put 2 tablespoons of olive oil in a pan over medium heat. Place the meatballs in the pan, approximately 2 inches apart from each other. Cook the meatballs for approximately 3 minutes on 1 side, then flip the meatballs onto the other side, and cook until lightly browned. Remove the cooked meatballs from the heat and repeat with the remaining meatballs. Once all of the meatballs have been pan-fried, add the grated carrots and zucchini to the pan and cook for 4 to 5 minutes. Add the jar of tomato sauce and cook for 10 minutes.

4. Place all of the meatballs back into the pan with the sauce. Simmer on low heat for 20 to 30 minutes. Serve the meatballs and sauce on top of the cooked pasta.

Grilled Portabella Mushroom Burger (With Sun-dried Tomato Yogurt Aioli)

Portabella Mushroom Burger

4 portabella mushrooms, washed and dried

4 whole wheat buns

2 cups baby spinach, washed and dried

Olive oil

SERVES
4

Asian Spice Marinade

1 teaspoon ground dried garlic (or 1 tablespoon fresh garlic)

2 bunches scallions, chopped

1 tablespoon sesame seeds

½ inch fresh ginger (or 1 teaspoon dried ginger)

½ cup soy sauce

Sun-dried Tomato Yogurt Aioli

1 garlic clove

10 sun-dried tomatoes (in oil)

¼ cup plain yogurt

2 tablespoons mayonnaise

Directions:

1. On a large baking tray, mix the marinade ingredients. Place the cleaned portabella mushrooms on the baking tray and let marinate for 30 minutes.

2. While the mushrooms are marinating, prepare the aioli. Put the garlic clove and sun-dried tomatoes in oil in a food processor and blend until smooth. Remove the mixture from the blender and place into a small bowl. Mix the yogurt and mayonnaise with the sun-dried tomato mixture until well blended.

3. Preheat a grill or large pan. If using a large pan, put 1 tablespoon of olive oil into the pan over medium heat. Once the pan or grill is heated, remove the mushrooms from the marinade and let cook for 5 minutes. Flip mushrooms onto the opposite side and let cook for another 3 to 4 minutes.

4. To prepare burgers, place 1 to 2 tablespoons of aioli on one side of the hamburger bun. Place the baby spinach on top of the aioli and then the mushroom on top of the spinach. Top the mushroom with the remaining hamburger bun and serve.

"Veggieful" Hamburgers

Ingredients:

1 pound lean ground beef or turkey

2 cups shredded vegetables
(carrots, zucchini, peppers)

½ cup uncooked oatmeal

1 teaspoon salt

½ teaspoon pepper

Whole wheat hamburger buns

Toppings: Lettuce, tomatoes, onions,
mushrooms, cheese

SERVES
4

Directions:

1. Mix the vegetables, meat, salt, pepper, and oatmeal in a bowl and stir. Take 2 large spoonfuls of the mixture and roll into a ball, then flatten to form a patty. Set the patty aside and repeat.

2. Put 1 tablespoon of olive oil in a pan over medium heat. Place the hamburger patties in the pan and cook for 5 to 6 minutes. Turn the patties over and cook for another 5 to 6 minutes. Serve the patties on hamburger buns with your favorite toppings!

Mexican Fiesta Stuffed Peppers

Ingredients:

4 bell peppers (any color)

1 cup crumbled feta cheese

1 15-ounce can black beans, drained

¼ cup cilantro, chopped

1 cup corn

2 cups cooked quinoa

1 tablespoon olive oil

SERVES
4

Directions:

Preheat the oven to 375°F. Cut the tops off the bell peppers and remove the seeds. Combine the remaining ingredients in a bowl and mix well. Divide the mixture evenly and stuff it into the peppers. Place the peppers in an ungreased baking pan and bake for 25 minutes. Serve with a side salad.

Smiling Faces Whole Wheat Pita Pizzas

SERVES 4

Ingredients:

4 loaves whole wheat pita
   bread

1 cup tomato sauce

2 cups assorted chopped vegetables
   (mushrooms, spinach, onions, peppers,
   broccoli)

1 cup shredded mozzarella cheese

Directions:

1. Preheat the oven to 400°F. Place 1 to 2 tablespoons of tomato sauce on each loaf of pita bread and spread evenly. Top the pita bread with vegetables and/or meat of your choice. (Encourage your kids to make a smiling face out of the toppings!) Sprinkle 2 tablespoons of cheese on top of the vegetables (or meat if you have any available). Place the pita loaves on an ungreased baking sheet and bake for 10 to 15 minutes, until the cheese is melted.

2. *Tip:* Make dessert pita pizzas! Slice ½ banana over each loaf of pita bread and sprinkle with 1 teaspoon of cinnamon. Bake at 400°F for 5 to 10 minutes. Remove the pita bread from the oven and drizzle 1 tablespoon of honey over each loaf.

Homemade Whole Wheat Rosemary Pizza

SERVES 6

Ingredients:

2 cups whole wheat flour

2 cups bread flour

2 teaspoons salt

2 tablespoons fresh rosemary,
   finely chopped

1¾ cups water, slightly warmer than
   room temperature

3 tablespoons olive oil

1 package rapidly rising yeast

2 cups mozzarella cheese

Lots of your favorite vegetables

Directions:

1. Place the water into a bowl and sprinkle in the yeast. Let the mixture sit for 4 to 5 minutes and then mix in the olive oil. Add the flours, salt, and rosemary, and mix with a wooden spoon. Knead by hand for approximately 10 minutes, ensuring the dough comes together. Place the dough in a large bowl and cover with a kitchen towel. Let the dough rise for 1½ to 2 hours, then uncover and see how much the dough has risen!

2. After the dough has risen, punch it down in the bowl. Divide the dough to make 6 individual pizzas. Roll out each piece on a well-floured surface. Spread tomato sauce on each pizza, sprinkle with cheese, and top with your favorite toppings. Bake on an ungreased baking sheet in the oven at 450°F for 12 to 15 minutes.

Eggplant Zucchini "Pasta" Lasagna

Eggplant Zucchini "Pasta"

1 large eggplant

3 medium zucchinis

1 24-ounce jar marinara sauce

1¼ cup low-fat mozzarella cheese

½ teaspoon salt

½ teaspoon pepper

SERVES
4

Italian Spice Marinade

1 teaspoon ground dried garlic (or 1 tablespoon fresh garlic)

1 teaspoon dried basil (or ¼ cup fresh basil, chopped)

1 teaspoon dried parsley (or ¼ cup fresh parsley, chopped)

1 teaspoon dried oregano

2 cups low-fat ricotta cheese

1 egg

Directions:

1. Preheat the oven to 400°F.

2. *To prepare the herbed ricotta:* In a bowl, mix the spices for the marinade. Mix in the ricotta and egg and stir well. Set aside.

3. *To prepare the vegetables:* Wash and dry the vegetables. Using a mandolin, slice the eggplant and zucchinis into thin strips lengthwise (mimicking the pasta used for lasagna). If you don't have a mandolin, carefully slice the eggplant and zucchinis lengthwise into very thin strips. Sprinkle the vegetable slices with salt and pepper and set aside.

4. *To assemble the lasagna:* Place ¼ cup of marinara sauce on the bottom of a 9 x 13-inch ungreased baking dish. Place a layer of zucchini/eggplant on top. Next, sprinkle a layer of mozzarella cheese, followed by a layer of the ricotta, and then a layer of marinara sauce. Place another layer of zucchini/eggplant and repeat the layers. Once complete, cover the baking dish with foil.

5. Bake for approximately 45 minutes. Remove the foil and sprinkle with ¼ cup of mozzarella cheese. Return the lasagna to the oven and bake for another 10 minutes, until the cheese has melted.

Whole Wheat Spinach Macaroni and Cheese

Ingredients:

½ pound whole wheat elbow macaroni

8 ounces frozen spinach, defrosted

4 cups skim milk

2 tablespoons butter

¼ cup all-purpose flour

1½ cups shredded cheddar cheese

1 teaspoon mustard

SERVES
4

Directions:

1. Cook the elbow macaroni according to package instructions. Drain the pasta after cooking and set aside. Melt the butter in a pot over medium heat. After the butter has melted, add the flour to the butter and continuously whisk to form a roux. Cook for 2 to 3 minutes and then slowly add the milk to the roux, continuously stirring while pouring the milk to make béchamel sauce Let cook for 5 to 7 minutes or until the béchamel sauce has thickened, stirring occasionally. Next, add the mustard and cheese. Cook for another 5 minutes, stirring occasionally, and then remove the pot from the heat.

2. Squeeze any excess water out of the defrosted spinach, add the spinach to the cooked pasta, and mix well. Pour the cheese sauce over the pasta, mix until well incorporated, and then serve.

Parmesan Crusted Baked Pasta

Ingredients:

1 pack whole wheat short pasta (penne, rigatoni, macaroni)

3 cups chopped assorted vegetables (such as broccoli, cauliflower, carrots, zucchini)

1 24-ounce jar of tomato or marinara sauce

1 cup grated Parmesan or mozzarella cheese

SERVES
6

Directions:

1. Cook the pasta as instructed on the label. Put 2 tablespoons of olive oil in a pan over medium heat. Place the vegetables in the pan and cook for 3 to 4 minutes, until the vegetables are tender. Pour the vegetables into a large mixing bowl and add the tomato/marinara sauce. Add the cooked pasta and stir. Pour the contents of the bowl into a large ungreased baking casserole dish.

2. Preheat the oven to 375°F. Place the casserole dish in the oven and bake for 30 minutes. Remove the dish from the oven and sprinkle cheese on top. Return the dish to the oven and bake another 15 minutes, until the cheese is melted.

Baked Egg Rolls

MAKES
8

Ingredients:

8 egg roll wrappers

2 carrots, peeled and grated

½ head green cabbage

1 9-ounce bag baby spinach

3 tablespoons soy sauce

½-inch piece fresh ginger

2 tablespoons olive oil

Directions:

1. *To prepare the vegetables:* Wash and dry all the vegetables. Chop the cabbage into thin slices and place the slices into a mixing bowl. Peel and grate the carrots and place them into the mixing bowl. Using the fine grating holes, grate the ginger and mix it in with the vegetables. Put olive oil in a pan over medium heat. Pour the vegetables from the mixing bowl into the pan and cook until the cabbage is soft, approximately 10 minutes. Add the spinach to the pan and stir. Once the spinach has wilted, add the soy sauce, stir, and remove the pan from the heat and let cool.

2. *To prepare the egg rolls:* Preheat the oven to 375°F. If the egg roll wrappers are square, arrange them so a diamond shape faces you. Dip your index finger in the water and paint the perimeter of the wrapper with water. Place 3 tablespoons of cooled vegetable filling in the center of the wrapper with more of the filling in the half of the wrapper closest to you. Fold in the left and right corners of the wrapper toward the filling. Then, fold the corner of the wrapper closest to you over the filling. Next, roll the covered filling toward the last corner and place the roll on an ungreased baking sheet in the baking sheet. With a pastry brush (or your index finger), lightly brush a thin layer of olive oil on both sides of the egg roll. Bake for approximately 15 minutes or until brown and crispy.

Whole Wheat Chow Mein

Ingredients:

SERVES
6

- 1 package whole wheat spaghetti, cooked
- 3 cups chopped assorted vegetables (mushrooms, spinach, peppers, carrots, snap peas)
- 1½ cups meat, sliced thin (chicken, pork, beef, or tofu)
- 1 medium onion, sliced
- 3 to 4 cloves of garlic, finely chopped
- 1-inch piece fresh ginger, finely chopped
- 1 cup green onions, chopped
- ¼ cup soy sauce
- 1 tablespoon honey

Directions:

Put 2 tablespoons of olive oil in a pan over medium heat. Place the onions, ginger, and garlic in the pan and cook for 3 to 4 minutes, stirring occasionally. Add the sliced meat to the pan and cook for 6 to 7 minutes or until the meat is almost cooked. Add the vegetables to the pan followed by the soy sauce and honey and cook for 2 minutes. Last, add the cooked noodles to the pan and mix all the ingredients well. Cook for another 2 to 3 minutes and then serve.

Cheesy Apple and Chard Quesadillas

Ingredients:

4 whole wheat tortillas

1 cup shredded cheddar cheese

1 large apple (any variety)

1 bunch Swiss chard

3 tablespoons olive oil

SERVES
4

Directions:

1. Wash and dry the Swiss chard, and then remove the leaves from the stems and discard the stems. Cut the Swiss chard into ribbons, approximately ¼-inch strips. Put 2 tablespoons of the olive oil in a pan over medium heat. Add the chard ribbons to the pan and cook for 4 to 5 minutes, until the chard has wilted. Remove the chard from the pan and wipe the pan clean. Drain the excess liquid from the cooked chard.

2. Wash the apple and cut it in half. Remove the core, and cut each piece in half again, lengthwise. Then, cut across each apple piece, making very thin slices.

3. To assemble the quesadillas, place ¼ cup of cheddar cheese on top of 1 tortilla. Place ½ cup of cooked chard in an even layer on top of the cheese. Next, place a single layer of apples on top of the chard. Sprinkle ¼ cup of cheddar cheese on top of the apples and cover with another tortilla. Repeat with remaining tortillas.

4. Put 1 tablespoon of olive oil in the pan over medium heat. Place 1 quesadilla in the pan and cook for 4 to 5 minutes. Flip the quesadilla over to the other side and cook for another 2 to 3 minutes. Serve with plain yogurt or guacamole.

Snacks and Dips

Yogurt Guacamole

SERVES
6

Ingredients:

3 ripe avocados

½ cup nonfat plain yogurt

1 garlic clove, finely chopped

¼ cup onion, finely chopped

¼ cup fresh cilantro, chopped

Juice of 1 lime

1 teaspoon salt

Directions:

In a bowl, mash the avocados well with a fork. Add the yogurt and mix well. Add the garlic, onion, cilantro, and stir. Mix in the lime juice and salt.

Creamy White Bean Hummus

Ingredients:

1 15-ounce can white beans
(also known as cannellini
beans), rinsed and drained

2 tablespoons olive oil

2 tablespoons water

1 clove garlic

Juice of ½ lemon

1 cucumber

Directions:

Blend beans, olive oil, water, garlic, and lemon juice in a blender until smooth. Cut the cucumber into ½-inch slices. To serve, dip raw vegetables into the hummus, or slice an English cucumber and top each slice with a dollop of hummus.

TIPS: Try adding different ingredients to the basic bean spread for new flavors.

★ Rosemary and sun-dried tomato dip: To previous ingredients, add 1 tablespoon of fresh rosemary and 5 to 6 sun-dried tomatoes.

★ Green onion and olive: To previous ingredients, add ¼ cup of chopped olives (seeds removed) and 1 bunch of green onions.

Five-Layer Bean Dip With Fresh Vegetables and Baked Pita Chips

Ingredients:

2 15-ounce cans black beans

6 tomatoes, seeded and chopped

2 ripe avocados

½ cup fresh cilantro, chopped

2 bunches green onions, chopped

½ cup cheddar cheese, shredded

1½ cups Greek yogurt

Juice of 1 lime

¼ medium white onion, finely chopped

Salt and pepper (to taste)

Directions:

1. *To prepare the beans:* Put the beans, including the water from the can, into a small pot over medium heat. Bring to a boil and then remove the pot from the heat. Using a fork or potato masher, mash the beans in the pot and then place them in an 8 x 8-inch baking dish.

2. *To prepare the guacamole*: Slice the avocado in half, remove the pit, and spoon the avocado into a bowl. Mix in the white onion and lime juice and sprinkle with salt and pepper. With a fork, mash the avocado with the onion and lime mixture. Then, add ¼ cup of Greek yogurt to the avocado mixture and mix well.

3. To assemble, spread the guacamole on top of the bean layer. Next, layer the chopped tomatoes on top of the guacamole. Spread the remainder of the Greek yogurt evenly on top of the tomatoes. Sprinkle the cheddar cheese on top of the yogurt, followed by the chopped cilantro and green onion.

4. Serve with fresh carrots, bell peppers, celery, cucumbers, or baked pita chips.

Baked Garlic Basil Pita Chips

Ingredients:

4 loaves whole wheat pita bread

3 tablespoons olive oil

½ teaspoon cayenne pepper

1 teaspoon garlic powder

1 teaspoon onion powder

2 teaspoons dried basil

1 teaspoon salt

Directions:

1. Preheat the oven to 400°F. In a bowl, mix the cayenne pepper, garlic powder, onion powder, basil, and salt with the olive oil. Cut each pita bread loaf into 4 pieces. Place the pita bread pieces on an ungreased baking sheet and drizzle with the spiced olive oil. Bake for 15 to 20 minutes, until the pita pieces are crisp.

2. Serve with hummus or as croutons for a salad.

TIP: Want a sweet twist? Instead of the noted spices, mix 1 tablespoon of cinnamon and 2 tablespoons of sugar and sprinkle over the pita bread. Bake 15 to 20 minutes, until the pita is crisp.

Crispy Spiced Chickpeas

Ingredients:

1 15-ounce can garbanzo beans (chickpeas)

2 tablespoons olive oil

1 teaspoon salt

½ teaspoon pepper

1 teaspoon cayenne pepper

1 teaspoon cumin

Directions:

Preheat the oven to 400°F. Drain the garbanzo beans through a colander and let them dry. After they are dry, put the garbanzo beans into a medium bowl, drizzle olive oil, and sprinkle spices over the beans. Mix well. Pour the beans onto an ungreased baking sheet and bake for 40 minutes, occasionally removing the sheet from the oven to stir the beans. Let cool and then serve.

Homemade Trail Mix Granola Bars

Ingredients:

1½ cups rolled oats

1½ cups crispy brown rice cereal

1 cup brown rice syrup

¼ cup brown sugar

1 cup whole or slivered almonds

1 cup raisins

½ cup chocolate chips

1 tablespoon ground cinnamon

1 teaspoon salt

2 tablespoons butter, melted and cooled

2 tablespoons flaxseed meal or flaxseeds (optional)

Directions:

Preheat the oven to 375°F. Mix all of the ingredients together in a mixing bowl. Spray a 9 x 13-inch pan with nonstick cooking spray. Pour the mixture into the baking pan and press the mixture down into the corners of the pan. Bake for 25 minutes. Cool to room temperature before cutting into bars.

Cinnamon Vanilla Yogurt "Fondue" With Apple Banana Kabobs

Ingredients:

1½ cups low-fat vanilla yogurt

1 tablespoon cinnamon

2 apples (any variety)

2 bananas

8 wooden skewers

Directions:

Place the yogurt and cinnamon into a bowl and mix well. Wash the apples, cut them into quarters, and remove the core. Slice each quarter across into 4 pieces/chunks and set aside. Peel the bananas and slice into ½-inch pieces. Place alternating pieces of the apples and bananas on the skewer. Serve with the yogurt "fondue." Remove the fruit from the skewers before serving to young children.

Dessert

Peanut Butter and Honey Crispy Squares

Ingredients:

½ cup peanut butter

½ cup honey

1 cup fiber cereal

2 tablespoons butter

Directions:

Mix the peanut butter, honey, and butter in a microwaveable bowl. Microwave on high for 45 seconds or until the peanut butter is melted. Mix in the cereal. Pour the mixture into a 9 x 13-inch pan and press the mixture into the corners of the pan. Let the mixture rest for 20 minutes and then cut it into squares.

Oatmeal Banana Chocolate Chip Cookies

Ingredients:

1 ripe banana

1 cup rolled oats

⅓ cup flaxseed meal

2 tablespoons
   olive oil

2 tablespoons maple syrup

½ teaspoon salt

2 teaspoons vanilla extract

⅓ cup chocolate chips

⅓ cup dried cherries

Directions:

Preheat the oven to 350°F. Mash the banana well and mix with the olive oil and vanilla extract. Mix the rolled oats, flaxseed meal, and salt with the banana mixture until well combined. Add in ⅓ cup of chocolate chips and ⅓ cup of dried cherries. Drop spoonfuls of the cookie dough on a greased baking sheet. Bake for approximately 12 minutes.

TIP: Try different combinations, such as dried cranberries and white chocolate or diced dried apples and butterscotch chips.

Frozen Chocolate Bananas

Ingredients:

2 bananas

½ cup chocolate chips

4 wooden skewers or popsicle sticks

¼ cup chopped nuts (optional)

Directions:

Peel the bananas and cut them in half. Insert a skewer through each banana half. Melt chocolate chips in the microwave and stir until the chocolate is smooth. Dip the bananas in the melted chocolate and place them on a baking sheet lined with foil. Sprinkle the bananas with nuts— if desired. Place the bananas in the freezer for at least 1 hour before serving.

Fruity Tropical Creamsicles

Ingredients:

2 cups plain nonfat yogurt

½ cup pineapple chunks

1 banana

1 orange, peeled and cut
    in half

½ cup mango chunks

½ cup strawberries

¼ cup honey

Small paper cups

Popsicle sticks

SERVES
4

Directions:

Place all the ingredients into a blender and blend until smooth. Pour the mixture into paper cups, and place a popsicle stick in the middle of each cup. Freeze overnight. To serve, peel the paper cups off of the popsicles and enjoy!

CarBaZu Muffins or Cupcakes

Ingredients:

1 cup oats

⅔ cup whole wheat flour

⅓ cup all-purpose flour

2 small carrots, peeled and grated

1 small zucchini, grated

1 ripe banana, mashed

⅔ cup buttermilk or plain yogurt

2 eggs

⅓ cup brown sugar

2 tablespoons unsalted butter, melted
  and cooled

1 teaspoon baking powder

1 teaspoon baking soda

½ teaspoon salt

2 teaspoons ground cinnamon

½ teaspoon ground nutmeg

SERVES
16

Directions:

1. Preheat the oven to 375°F. Lightly beat the eggs in a medium mixing bowl. Add the yogurt (or buttermilk) to the eggs and stir. Add the cooled butter to the wet ingredients and then add the brown sugar and stir the mixture. Squeeze any excess water out of the grated zucchini. Mix the grated carrots, zucchini, and mashed bananas into the wet ingredients.

2. For the dry ingredients, place the oats in a blender and blend until a fine powder. Pour the oat flour into a mixing bowl and add the whole wheat and all-purpose flours. Mix in the baking soda, baking powder, and salt. Stir the cinnamon and nutmeg into the flour mixture.

3. Pour half of the flour mixture into the wet ingredients and gently stir. Add the remainder of the flour mixture and mix gently until well incorporated. Pour the batter into lined muffin tins, about ⅔ full. Bake for 20 minutes.

TIP: Transform the muffin into a cupcake with a dollop of honey cream cheese frosting (recipe on next page).

Honey Cream Cheese Frosting

Ingredients:

1 8-ounce package light cream cheese, room temperature

¼ cup honey

1 tablespoon cinnamon

Directions:

Use an electric mixer to mix together all of the ingredients. Put a dollop of the mixture on top of a muffin to make a cupcake.

Quick Graham Cracker Apple Crisp

Ingredients:

2 apples (any variety)

¼ cup brown sugar

1 tablespoon cinnamon

1 teaspoon nutmeg

1 tablespoon lemon juice

6 graham crackers

¼ cup pecans, chopped

2 tablespoons butter, melted

SERVES
4

Directions:

1. Slice the apples in half and core them. Then, slice the apple halves horizontally in half, resulting in 4 total pieces. Next, slice the apple pieces across into ¼-inch chunks and place in a large mixing bowl. Add the brown sugar, cinnamon, nutmeg, lemon juice, and half of the melted butter. Mix well and pour the mixture into a microwaveable dish.

2. For the topping, crush the graham crackers into crumbs and pour them into a bowl. Add the pecans and remaining butter to the bowl and stir. Sprinkle the graham cracker/pecan topping onto the apples and microwave on high for 10 to 12 minutes. Serve with a dollop of low-fat vanilla yogurt.

Reinforcement Planners

Family SWOT Analysis
(Figure 1.1 in Chapter 1)

S	W	O	T
Strengths	**Weaknesses**	**Opportunities**	**Threats**

General Functioning Subscale of the McMaster Family Assessment Device
(Figure 1.2 in Chapter 1)

	Strongly Agree	Agree	Disagree	Strongly Disagree
1. Planning family activities is difficult because we misunderstand each other.	4	3	2	1
2. In time of crisis we can turn to each other for support.	1	2	3	4
3. We cannot talk to each other about sadness we feel.	4	3	2	1
4. Individuals are accepted for what they are.	1	2	3	4
5. We avoid discussing our fears and concerns.	4	3	2	1
6. We can express feelings to each other.	1	2	3	4
7. There are lots of bad feelings in the family.	4	3	2	1
8. We feel accepted for what we are.	1	2	3	4
9. Making decisions is a problem for our family.	4	3	2	1
10. We are able to make decisions about how to solve problems.	1	2	3	4
11. We don't get along well together.	4	3	2	1
12. We confide in each other.	1	2	3	4

Scoring

The questionnaire is scored by summing the numbers for each box you checked in questions 1 through 12. Then divide the sum by 12. Scores range from 1.0 (best functioning) to 4.0 (worst functioning).

If you find that there are areas for improvement, come up with a plan for how you might function better. If you find that there are many challenges, or it is difficult to come up with a plan to get along better, you might consider reaching out to a professional who specializes in helping families thrive.

Source: Used with permission by Epstein NB, Baldwin LM, Bishop DS. The McMaster Family Assessment Device. *J Marital Fam Ther.* 1983;9(2):171–180.

Previsit Checklist
(Figure 1.3 in Chapter 1)

	Things I Do Well as a Parent	Things I Would Like to Discuss Today
Feeding my child		
Understanding what to expect next from my child		
Managing my child's behavior		
Helping my child sleep		
Using resources in my community to help my child		
Helping my child fit into our family; get along with others		
Helping my family handle stress		
Helping my child learn through play and be physically active		
Managing my child's moods		
Managing my child's screen time		
Setting routines		

Source: Adapted from American Academy of Pediatrics. *Bright Futures: Nutrition.* Elk Grove Village, IL: American Academy of Pediatrics; 2011.

How Connected Are You to Your Community?
(Figure 1.7 in Chapter 1)

	Not at all	Somewhat	Mostly	Completely
I can trust people in this community.				
I can recognize most of the members of this community.				
Most community members know me.				
This community has symbols and expressions of membership such as clothes, signs, art, architecture, logos, landmarks, and flags that people can recognize.				
I put a lot of time and effort into being part of this community.				
Being a member of this community is a part of my identity.				
It is very important to me to be a part of this community.				
I am with other community members a lot and enjoy being with them.				
I expect to be a part of this community for a long time.				
Members of this community have shared important events together, such as holidays, celebrations, or disasters.				
I feel hopeful about the future of this community.				
Members of this community care about each other.				
My community can work together to improve its health.				
My community has the resources to improve its health.				
My community works together to make positive change for health.				
I know my neighbors will help me stay healthy.				

Source: Adapted with permission from RAND. Well-Being 425—Culture of Health.
https://alpdata.rand.org/index.php?page=data&p=showsurvey&syid=425. Accessed July 1, 2019.

Making Sense of Your Photo Food Log
(Figure 2.2 in Chapter 2)

	Breakfast	Lunch	Dinner	Snack	Total
Fruit 1 cup-equiv of fruit is: • 1 cup of raw or cooked fruit • ½ cup of dried fruit • 1 cup of 100% fruit juice					(cups)
Vegetables 1 cup-equiv of vegetables is: • 1 cup of raw or cooked vegetables • 2 cups of leafy salad greens • 1 cup of 100% vegetable juice					(cups)
Protein 1 ounce-equiv of protein is: • 1 ounce of lean meat, poultry, or seafood • 1 egg • 1 tablespoon of peanut butter • ¼ cup of cooked beans or peas • ½ ounce of nuts or seeds					(ounces)
Grains 1 ounce-equiv of grains is: • 1 slice of bread • 1 ounce of ready-to-eat cereal • ½ cup of cooked rice, pasta, or cereal					(ounces)
Dairy/Substitute 1 cup-equiv of dairy is: • 1 cup of milk • 1 cup of yogurt • 1 cup of fortified soy beverage • 1½ ounces of natural cheese or 2 ounces of processed cheese					(cups)

Keeping Tabs on Physical Activity
(Figure 2.4 in Chapter 2)

Family Member	Mon	Tues	Wed	Thurs	Fri	Sat	Sun

**Fitness Assessment Log
(Figure 2.5 in Chapter 2)**

Date:

Family Member	1 Mile Time	Crunches (total in 2 min)	Push-ups/ Modified Push-ups (total in 2 min)	Shoulder Stretch Distance Right (R) Left (L)	Waist Circumference (inches)	Height (ft, in)	Weight (lb)	BMI (number for adult or % for child/ adolescent)[a]

Abbreviation: BMI, body mass index.

[a] BMI is height (in meters)/weight (in kg). Use the Centers for Disease Control and Prevention BMI calculator to determine BMI for adults and BMI percentiles for children and teens (http://cdc.gov/BMI).

Sleep Logs
Adults Tracker
(Figure 2.6 from Chapter 2)

⬥ NATIONAL SLEEP FOUNDATION

SLEEP LOG: Please fill this out for the previous day and night no more than 3 hours after waking. The information can be an estimate when necessary. This sleep log is provided by the National Sleep Foundation, www.sleepfoundation.org.

NAME _____   WEEK OF _____

DAY	Sun	Mon	Tues	Wed	Thurs	Fri	Sat
1. Did you nap? a. For how long? b. At what time?	Yes No _____min	Yes No _____min	Yes No _____min	Yes No _____min	Yes No _____min	Yes No _____min	Yes No _____min
2. Did you have any caffeine* after 6pm?	Yes No	Yes No	Yes No	Yes No	Yes No	Yes No	Yes No
3. Did you drink alcohol after 6pm?	Yes No	Yes No	Yes No	Yes No	Yes No	Yes No	Yes No
4. Did you use nicotine after 6pm?	Yes No	Yes No	Yes No	Yes No	Yes No	Yes No	Yes No
5. Did you exercise?	Yes No	Yes No	Yes No	Yes No	Yes No	Yes No	Yes No
6. Did you eat a heavy meal or snack after 6pm?	Yes No	Yes No	Yes No	Yes No	Yes No	Yes No	Yes No
7. Did you take any sleeping medication a. What medication? b. Amount c. At what time?	Yes No	Yes No	Yes No	Yes No	Yes No	Yes No	Yes No
8. Were you sleepy during the day?	Yes No	Yes No	Yes No	Yes No	Yes No	Yes No	Yes No
NIGHT							
1. What time did you turn off the lights to go to sleep?							
2. What time did you wake up?							
3. How many total hours did you sleep?							
4. How many times did you wake up in the night?							
5. Rate the quality of your sleep: 1=poor, 5=excellent							
6. Do you feel you got enough sleep?							

Caffeine = coffee, tea, caffeinated soda, chocolate, energy drinks, certain medications.

Reprinted with permission from https://sleepfoundation.org/sites/default/files/
sample_sleep_log-by_national_sleep_foundation.pdf

Sleep Logs *(continued)*
Kids Tracker
(Figure 2.6 from Chapter 2)

Day	Sun	Mon	Tues	Wed	Thurs	Fri	Sat
How was your child's mood and energy during the day? (good, OK, bad)							
How well did your child pay attention at school or home? (not at all, OK, great)							
Did your child take a nap? If yes, when and for how long?							
Did your child consume any caffeine (eg, soda, chocolate, tea)? If yes, at what time?							
Did your child exercise? If yes, when and for how long?							
Did your child use a screen (eg, TV, tablet, phone) within 1 hour of bedtime?							
Did your child follow a bedtime routine? If yes, what?							
Night	**Sun**	**Mon**	**Tues**	**Wed**	**Thurs**	**Fri**	**Sat**
What time did your child go to bed?							
How easily did your child fall asleep?							
How many times did your child wake in the night?							
How many total hours did your child sleep?							
Was your child disturbed by any noise, lights, temperature, sound, nightmares, stress, pain, hunger, thirst, etc? If so, by what?							
When your child woke for the day, was s/he well rested?							

Adapted with permission from http://www.sleepforkids.org/pdf/SleepDiary.pdf

How Do You Cope With Stress?
(Figure 2.7 in Chapter 2)

Example	I do this a lot.	I do not do this a lot.	Type of Coping
I do something to think about it less, such as going to movies, watching TV, reading, daydreaming, sleeping, shopping [or exercising].			Self-distraction (A)
I take action to try to make the situation better.			Active coping (A)
I say to myself, "This isn't real."			Denial (M)
I use alcohol or other drugs [or food] to make myself feel better.			Substance use (M)
I get emotional support from others.			Use of emotional support (A)
I get help and advice from other people.			Instrumental support (A)
I give up the attempt to cope.			Behavioral disengagement (M)
I say things to let my unpleasant feelings escape.			Venting (M)
I look for something good in what is happening.			Positive reframing (A)
I try to come up with a strategy about what to do.			Planning (A)
I make jokes about it.			Humor (A)
I accept the reality of the fact that it has happened.			Acceptance (A)
I pray or meditate.			Religion/spirituality (A)
I blame myself for things that happened.			Self-blame (M)

Abbreviations: A, adaptive, or generally helpful coping strategy; M, maladaptive, or generally unhelpful coping strategy.

Adapted with permission from Springer Nature Customer Service Centre GmbH: Springer Nature. Carver CS. You want to measure coping but your protocol's too long: consider the brief COPE. *Int J Behav Med*. 1997;4(1):92–100

Your Family Fit Plan
(Figure 3.7 in Chapter 3)

THE _____ FAMILY FIT PLAN

Our "Why":

Our Vision:

		SMART Goal 1	Action 1	Action 2	Action 3
Nutrition		SMART Goal 2	Action 1	Action 2	Action 3
		SMART Goal 3	Action 1	Action 2	Action 3
Physical activity		SMART Goal 1	Action 1	Action 2	Action 3
		SMART Goal 2	Action 1	Action 2	Action 3
		SMART Goal 3	Action 1	Action 2	Action 3
Sleep		SMART Goal 1	Action 1	Action 2	Action 3
		SMART Goal 2	Action 1	Action 2	Action 3
		SMART Goal 3	Action 1	Action 2	Action 3

(continued)

Your Family Fit Plan (continued)
(Figure 3.7 in Chapter 3)

	SMART Goal 1	Action 1	Action 2	Action 3
Screen time				
	SMART Goal 2	Action 1	Action 2	Action 3
	SMART Goal 3	Action 1	Action 2	Action 3
Stress management	SMART Goal 1	Action 1	Action 2	Action 3
	SMART Goal 2	Action 1	Action 2	Action 3
	SMART Goal 3	Action 1	Action 2	Action 3

Weekly Meal Planner
(Figure 4.1 in Chapter 4)

	Sun	Mon	Tue	Wed	Thu	Fri	Sat
Breakfast							
Lunch							
Dinner							
Snacks							
Notes							

The Family Fit Tracker
(Figure 5.2 in Chapter 5)

HEALTH TRACKER

MONTH/YEAR: _____

		FOOD	PHYSICAL ACTIVITY
MONDAY	B		
	L		
	D		
	S		
TUESDAY	B		
	L		
	D		
	S		
WEDNESDAY	B		
	L		
	D		
	S		
THURSDAY	B		
	L		
	D		
	S		
FRIDAY	B		
	L		
	D		
	S		
SATURDAY	B		
	L		
	D		
	S		
SUNDAY	B		
	L		
	D		
	S		

Taste Test! Dips
(LET'S EXPERIMENT Box in Chapter 5)

Vegetable	Before Rating	Raw Rating	Dip 1 (Creamy White Bean Hummus)	Dip 2 (Rosemary and Sun-dried Tomato)	Dip 3 (Green Onion and Olive)

Your Family Then. Your Family Now.
(Mindful Moment Box in Chapter 7)

	Then	Now
Nutrition		
Physical activity		
Sleep		
Stress management		
Screen time		

Workouts

*Make sure you warm up
for 2 to 3 minutes
before each workout
and cool down for
2 to 3 minutes
after each workout.*

High-Intensity Aerobic Interval Walking

High-intensity aerobic interval walking consists of up to 10 high-intensity walking intervals lasting 4 minutes each, interspersed with 2-minute relief-walking intervals.

Walk as fast as you can (hard to very hard intensity) for 4 minutes and then walk at an easy pace for the next 2 minutes. Repeat.

Start with shorter high-intensity intervals (2 minutes or even 1 minute) and rest periods. As your fitness improves, gradually increase the time and number of intervals you complete.

Sprint Interval Walking

Sprint-walk as fast as you can for 30 seconds.

Then "rest" with 4 minutes 30 seconds of light walking. Repeat 4 times.

3-Minute Jump Rope Workout

All you need is a jump rope and a timer.

Basic jump—30 seconds

Side to side—30 seconds

Single leg right—30 seconds

Single leg left—30 seconds

Backward or basic jump repeat—30 seconds

Alternating foot—30 seconds

The 7-Minute Workout

Each interval is 30 seconds, separated by 10 seconds of rest. You can time it yourself or use one of the many available 7-minute workout apps.

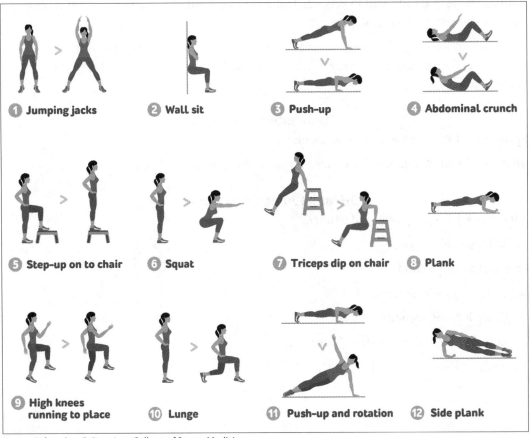

1. Jumping jacks
2. Wall sit
3. Push-up
4. Abdominal crunch
5. Step-up on to chair
6. Squat
7. Triceps dip on chair
8. Plank
9. High knees running to place
10. Lunge
11. Push-up and rotation
12. Side plank

Source [of workout]: American College of Sports Medicine

Animal-Inspired Yoga

Yoga is an activity that anyone can learn to do, even toddlers! Start with these 4 animal-inspired yoga poses to help your family slow down, de-stress, and improve muscular strength and endurance, all at the same time!

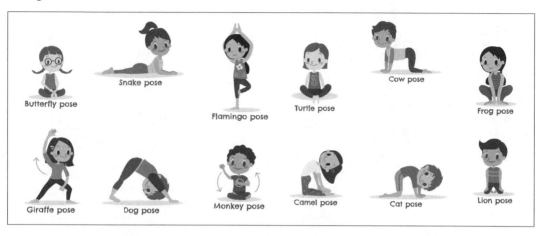

Yoga Sun Salutations for Beginners

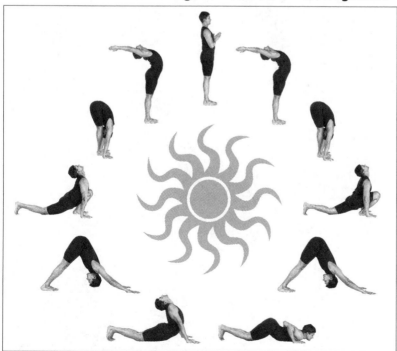

Create a lasting memory with your child while getting fit by completing the yoga sun salutations sequence for beginners. Engage all of your senses by playing soft music, lighting an aromatic candle, and taking deep mindful breaths while you go through the sequence.

Source of workout: https://www.acefitness.org/education-and-resources/lifestyle/blog/6835/a-beginner-s-guide-to-sun-salutations

Resources

Many resources are available to help your family achieve your fitness and health goals. Here are a few from the American Academy of Pediatrics (AAP).

Achieving a Healthy Weight for Your Child: An Action Plan for Families

by Sandra G. Hassink, MD, MS, FAAP: This book helps parents of children affected by overweight or obesity.

Bright Futures Resources for Families

(https://brightfutures.aap.org/families/Pages/Resources-for-Families.aspx): This site provides links to developmentally tailored messages and resources that help support your child's growth and development.

Healthy Growth app

(https://www.aap.org/en-us/Pages/Get-the-AAP-Mobile-App.aspx): This app provides parents with information to support healthy growth, nutrition, and physical activity for children 5 years and younger.

Institute for Healthy Childhood Weight

(https://ihcw.aap.org): The institute provides information and tools to families, pediatricians, and policy makers to better prevent and treat childhood obesity.

The Picky Eater Project: 6 Weeks to Happier, Healthier Family Mealtimes

by Natalie Digate Muth, MD, MPH, RDN, FAAP, and Sally Sampson: This book helps parents undo picky eating. Recipes from this book are available at www.HealthyChildren.org/recipes.

References

Chapter 1

1. Harper Browne C. The Strengthening Families Approach and Protective Factors Framework: Branching out and reaching deeper. 2014; https://www.cssp.org/reform/strengtheningfamilies/2014/The-Strengthening-Families-Approach-and-Protective-Factors-Framework_Branching-Out-and-Reaching-Deeper.pdf. Accessed October 19, 2018

2. American Academy of Pediatrics. Eliciting parental strengths and needs. *Bright Futures Implementation Tip Sheet* 2015; https://brightfutures.aap.org/Bright%20Futures%20Documents/AAP_BF_ElicitingParentalStrength_Tipsheet_FINAL.pdf. Accessed October 11, 2018

3. American Academy of Pediatrics. *Bright Futures, Nutrition*. Elk Grove Village, IL: American Academy of Pediatrics; 2011

4. Centers for Disease Control and Prevention. https://www.cdc.gov/healthyweight/assessing/bmi/childrens_bmi/about_childrens_bmi.html. Accessed March 19, 2019

5. Adolescent Sleep Working Group, Committee on Adolescence, and Council on School Health. Policy statement: School start times for adolescents. *Pediatrics*. 2014;134(3):642–649

6. Robert Wood Johnson Foundation. National Survey of Health Attitudes. 2015; https://www.rwjf.org/en/cultureofhealth/taking-action/making-health-a-shared-value/sense-of-community.html. Accessed October 11, 2018

7. RAND. Well Being 425—Culture of Health. https://alpdata.rand.org/index.php?page=data&p=showsurvey&syid=425. Accessed July 1, 2019

Chapter 4

1. Pollan M. *In Defense of Food: An Eater's Manifesto*. New York, NY: The Penguin Group; 2008

2. Pollan M. Rules to eat by. 2009; https://michaelpollan.com/articles-archive/rules-to-eat-by/. Accessed September 29, 2018

3. Baumrind D. Current patterns of parental authority. *Developmental Psychology Monograph*. 1971;4((1, Part 2)):1–101

4. Hohman EE, Paul IM, Birch LL, Savage JS. INSIGHT responsive parenting intervention is associated with healthier patterns of dietary exposures in infants. *Obesity (Silver Spring)*. 2017;25(1):185–191

5. Vedanthan R, Bansilal S, Soto AV, et al. Family-based approaches to cardiovascular health promotion. *J Am Coll Cardiol*. 2016;67(14):1725–1737

6. United States Department of Agriculture. MyPlate. https://choosemyplate.gov. Accessed April 1, 2019

7. Muth ND, Sampson S. *The Picky Eater Project: 6 Weeks to Happier, Healthier Family Mealtimes*. Elk Grove Village, IL: American Academy of Pediatrics; 2016:51

8. Dallacker M, Hertwig R, Mata J. The frequency of family meals and nutritional health in children: a meta-analysis. *Obes Rev*. 2018;19(5):638–653

9. Duke MP, Lazarus A, Fivush R. Knowledge of family history as a clinically useful index of psychological well-being and prognosis: A brief report. *Psychotherapy (Chic)*. 2008;45(2):268–272

10. Advice. Top Table Manners for Kids. What Every Kid Should Know. The Emily Post Institute. http://emilypost.com/advice/top-table-manners-for-kids/. Accessed March 7, 2019

11. Orlet Fisher J, Rolls BJ, Birch LL. Children's bite size and intake of an entree are greater with large portions than with age-appropriate or self-selected portions. *Am J Clin Nutr*. 2003;77(5):1164–1170

Chapter 5

1. Goyal M, Singh S, Sibinga EM, et al. Meditation programs for psychological stress and well-being: a systematic review and meta-analysis. *JAMA Intern Med*. 2014;174(3):357–368

2. Johnson SL. Improving preschoolers' self-regulation of energy intake. *Pediatrics*. 2000;106(6):1429–1435

3. Orlet Fisher J, Rolls BJ, Birch LL. Children's bite size and intake of an entree are greater with large portions than with age-appropriate or self-selected portions. *Am J Clin Nutr*. 2003;77(5):1164–1170

4. Gillen JB, Martin BJ, MacInnis MJ, Skelly LE, Tarnopolsky MA, Gibala MJ. Twelve weeks of sprint interval training improves indices of cardiometabolic health similar to traditional endurance training despite a five-fold lower exercise volume and time commitment. *PLoS One*. 2016;11(4):e0154075

5. Rolls BJ, Engell D, Birch LL. Serving portion size influences 5-year-old but not 3-year-old children's food intakes. *J Am Diet Assoc*. 2000;100(2):232–234

6. Tanofsky-Kraff M, Haynos AF, Kotler LA, Yanovski SZ, Yanovski JA. Laboratory-based studies of eating among children and adolescents. *Curr Nutr Food Sci*. 2007;3(1):55–74

7. Ray A. https://amitray.com/amitray_quotes/. Accessed March 8, 2019

8. Seligman ME, Csikszentmihalyi M. Positive psychology. An introduction. *Am Psychol*. 2000;55(1):5–14

Chapter 6

1. Vos MB, Kaar JL, Welsh JA, et al. Added sugars and cardiovascular disease risk in children: a scientific statement from the American Heart Association. *Circulation.* 2017;135(19):e1017–e1034

2. Jiang J. How teens and parents navigate screen time and device distractions. Pew Research Center website. http://www.pewinternet.org/2018/08/22/how-teens-and-parents-navigate-screen-time-and-device-distractions. Published August 22, 2018. Accessed March 18, 2019

3. Anderson M, Jiang J. Teens, social media & technology 2018. Pew Research Center website. http://www.pewinternet.org/2018/05/31/teens-social-media-technology-2018. Published May 31, 2018. Accessed March 18, 2019

4. Nestle M. Food marketing and childhood obesity—a matter of policy. *N Engl J Med.* 2006;354(24):2527–2529

5. Boyland E, Whalen R, Christiansen P, et al. *See It, Want It, Buy It, Eat It: How Food Advertising Is Associated With Unhealthy Eating Behaviors in 7–11 Year Old Children.* Cancer Research UK. https://www.cancerresearchuk.org/sites/default/files/see_it_want_it_buy_it_eat_it_final_report.pdf. Published October 2018. Accessed March 18, 2019

6. McGinnis J, Gootman JA, Kraak VI. *Food Marketing to Children and Youth: Threat or Opportunity?* Washington, DC: The National Academies Press; 2006

7. Veerman JL, Van Beeck EF, Barendregt JJ, Mackenbach JP. By how much would limiting TV food advertising reduce childhood obesity? *Eur J Public Health.* 2009;19(4):365–369

8. Buijzen M, Valkenburg PM. The effects of television advertising on materialism, parent–child conflict, and unhappiness: a review of research. *Appl Dev Psychol.* 2003;24(4):437–456

9. Bragg MA, Miller AN, Elizee J, Dighe S, Elbel BD. Popular music celebrity endorsements in food and nonalcoholic beverage marketing. *Pediatrics.* 2016;138(1):e20153977

10. Lapierre MA, Vaala SE, Linebarger DL. Influence of licensed spokescharacters and health cues on children's ratings of cereal taste. *Arch Pediatr Adolesc Med.* 2011;165(3):229–234

11. Coates AE, Hardman CA, Halford JCG, Christiansen P, Boyland EJ. Social medial infuencer marketing and children's food intake: a randomized controlled trial. *Pediatrics.* 2019;143(4):e20182554

12. Sims J, Mikkelsen L, Gibson P, Warming E. *Claiming Health: Front-of-package Labeling of Children's Food.* Oakland, CA: Prevention Institute; 2011

13. Trasande L, Shaffer RM, Sathyanarayana S; American Academy of Pediatrics Council on Environmental Health. Food additives and child health. *Pediatrics.* 2018;142(2):e20181408

14. Mikkelsen L, Merlo C, Lee V, Chao C. *Where's the Fruit? Fruit Content of the Most Highly-Advertised Children's Food and Beverages.* Oakland, CA: Prevention Institute; 2007

Chapter 7

1. Baumeister RF, Bratslavsky, E, Finkenauer C, Vohs KD. Bad is stronger than good. *Rev Gen Psychol.* 2001;5(4):323–370

2. Bryant FB, Veroff J. *Savoring: A New Model of Positive Experience.* Mahwah, NJ: Lawrence Erlbaum Associates; 2007

3. Wood AM, Froh JJ, Geraghty AW. Gratitude and well-being: a review and theoretical integration. *Clin Psychol Rev.* 2010;30(7):890–905

4. Froh JJ, Sefick WJ, Emmons RA. Counting blessings in early adolescents: an experimental study of gratitude and subjective well-being. *J Sch Psychol.* 2008;46(2):213–233

5. Froh JJ, Fan J, Emmons RA, Bono G, Huebner ES, Watkins P. Measuring gratitude in youth: assessing the psychometric properties of adult gratitude scales in children and adolescents. *Psychol Assess.* 2011;23(2):311–324

6. Jackson SA, Marsh HW. Development and validation of a scale to measure optimal experience: the Flow State Scale. *J Sport Exerc Psychol.* 1996;18(1):17–35

7. Csikszentmihalyi M, Rathune K, Whalen S. *Talented Teenagers: The Roots of Success and Failure.* Cambridge, UK: Cambridge University Press; 1997

Chapter 8

1. Leung AWY, Chan RSM, Sea MMM, Woo J. An overview of factors associated with adherence to lifestyle modification programs for weight management in adults. *Int J Environ Res Public Health.* 2017;14(8):E922

2. Van Horn L, Carson JA, Appel LJ, et al; American Heart Association Nutrition Committee of the Council on Lifestyle and Cardiometabolic Health, Council on Cardiovascular Disease in the Young, Council on Cardiovascular and Stroke Nursing, Council on Clinical Cardiology, and Stroke Council. Recommended dietary pattern to achieve adherence to the American Heart Association/American College of Cardiology (AHA/ACC) guidelines: a scientific statement from the American Heart Association. *Circulation.* 2016;134(22):e505–e529

3. Nicklas TA, Jahns L, Bogle ML, et al. Barriers and facilitators for consumer adherence to the Dietary Guidelines for Americans: the HEALTH study. *J Acad Nutr Diet.* 2013;113(10):1317–1331

4. Lemstra M, Bird Y, Nwankwo C, Rogers M, Moraros J. Weight loss intervention adherence and factors promoting adherence: a meta-analysis. *Patient Prefer Adherence.* 2016;10:1547–1559

Index

Page numbers followed by *f* indicate a figure.

DEC - - 2019